CODE GREEN

HIDDEN POWERS OF THE GARDEN
TARGETING THE IMMUNE SYSTEM

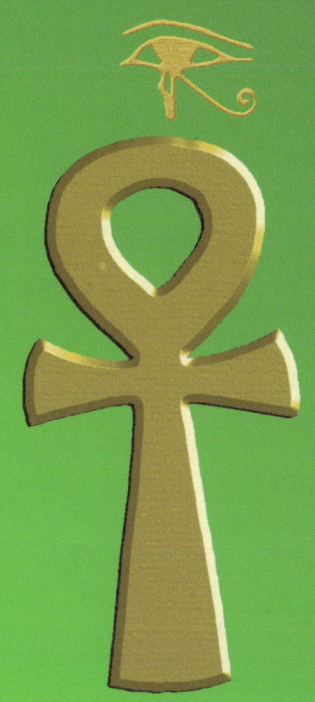

HIGH PRIEST KWATAMANI
KWATAMANI FIRST GENESIS TRIBE

visuals, juicing, sprouting, recipes

**Published by the Kwatamani Holistic Institute of
Brain Body & Spiritual Research & Dev., Inc.**

Email: kwatamani@earthlink.net
kwatamani@livefoodsunchild.com
Website: http://www.livefoodsunchild.com
http://www.Kwa-Ta-Man-I-Temple.org

Editors:
High Priest Kwatamani
and the Kwatamani Royal Family
**Feminine-Energy Translator and Researcher
for the High Priest Kwatamani:**
Senior Royal Priestess KwaNanaMu Kwatamani,
Editing Coordinator and
Spiritual Ɔkyame of the Queen Mother
and the Kwatamani Royal Sisterhood
Technical Editor: KwaMasu Kwatamani

MANIFESTING THE EXPRESSIONS OF
SUPREME LOVE, RIGHTEOUSNESS &
THE HOLISTIC LIVING TRUTH
ABOUT SUPREME LOVE

First Edition
Release Date: May, 2020
Copyright © 2020. All rights reserved.

TABLE OF CONTENTS

- Opening Song: "As It Was in the Beginning" — 6
- Introduction: Let Food Be Your Medicine — 9
- Chapter 1: Strengthening Immunity — 11
  - Holistic Living Survival — 11
  - Life Sustaining Fueling Source — 12
  - Why Nutrition is Key — 15
  - Viruses, Bacteria, Protozoa & Fungi — 16
  - Antibodies: Building Defense — 17
  - Immune System Fundamentals — 17
  - Nutritional Support Is a Must — 19
- Chapter 2: Antioxidants & Micronutrients from A to Z — 21
  - Vitamin A — 22
  - Special Focus: Nutritional Protection (Vitamin A, Vitamin B-complex, Vitamin C, Vitamin D, Vitamin E, and Zinc) — 24
  - Vitamin B — 25
  - Vitamin C — 26
  - Vitamin D and Vitamin E — 28
  - Zinc — 31
- Chapter 3: Did You Eat Your Greens? — 33
  - Kale — 34
  - Cruciferous Vegetables — 37

- Lettuce — 40
- Chapter 4: The Best Defense (Fresh from the Garden) — 43
- Chapter 5: Back to the Basics — 47
  - Super Foods: Coconuts — 48
  - Super Foods: Tomatoes — 50
  - Super Foods: Celery — 52
  - Super Foods: Bell Peppers — 53
  - Super Foods: Garlic — 54
  - Super Foods: Onion — 55
- Chapter 6: Juicing & Sprouting — 57
  - Juicing — 58
  - Go Green Immunity Tonic — 61
  - Red Alert Immunity Tonic — 63
  - Immuno-Green Super Soup — 64
- Chapter 7: Raw Vegan Dishes – Green Immuno Fuel — 69
  - Marinated Mixed Greens — 70
  - Popular Island Bush Greens: Callaloo — 72
  - Sesame Seed Supreme — 74
  - Cabbage Sammich with Brazil Nut Loaf — 78
  - Okra in the Raw — 85
  - Chia Fruit Pudding — 89
  - Kemetic Kush Supreme: Kwa-Touli#9 — 93
- Chapter 8: Herbal Defense -- Culinary Condiments — 97
  - Basil, cilantro, culantro, dill — 98
  - Garlic, ginger, lemongrass, mint — 99

TABLE OF CONTENTS

- ○ Onion, oregano, parsley — 100
- ○ Peppers — 101
- ○ Rosemary, thyme, turmeric — 102
- Chapter 9: Environmental Immunity — 105
  - ○ Depleting and Devitalizing — 106
  - ○ First Genesis — 109
- Closing Song: "A New Day Has Begun" — 114

Opening Song: "As It Was in the Beginning"

Senior Priestess KwaNanamu Kwatamani and the Sacred Ancestral Naga Priestesses

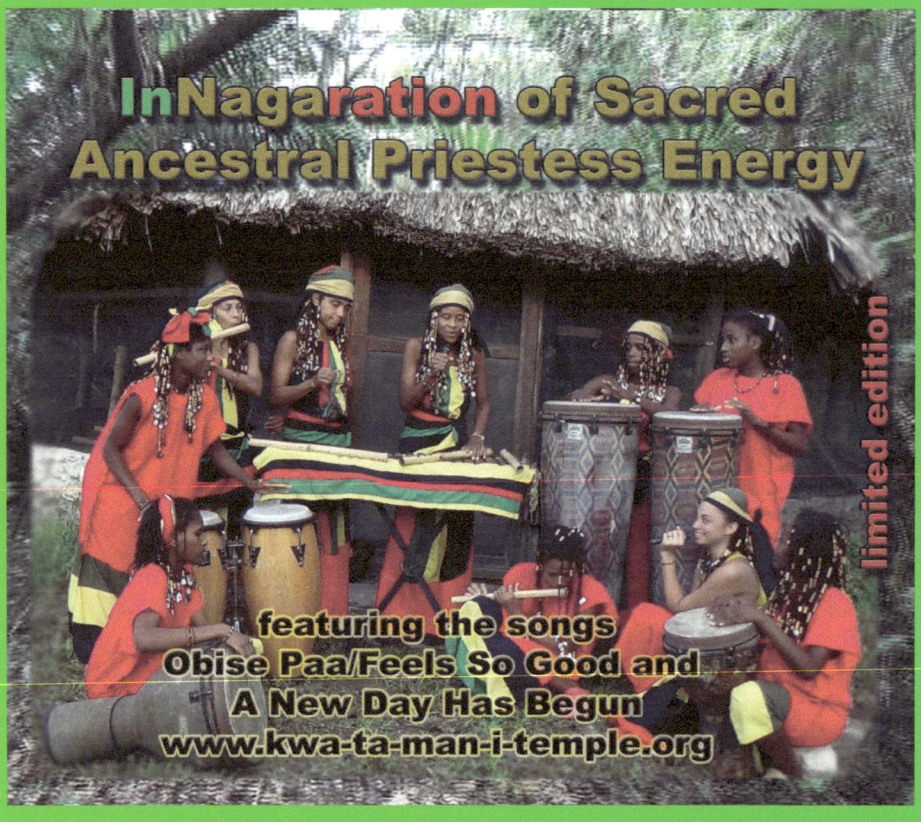

Released November 2014
Sacred Ancestral Temple of Kwa-Ta-Man-I
Kemetic Naga Priesthood

Sacred Garden Culture, culture
Divine Children of the Sun, sun
As it was in the beginning,
in the beginning
A new day has begun

People get ready,
The Sacred Ancestral Naga Priesthood has come
the Sacred Ancestral Naga Priesthood has come
Sacred Garden Culture
Divine Children of the Sun
As it was in the beginning
A new day has begun
People get ready, there's a change a coming
People get ready, the Sacred Ancestral Naga Priesthood has come

Divine intervention of the Most High Plan
The Most Supreme Unseen said "Let us make Man"
Oh, Man, He and She, came to the Earth divinely
He and She, came to the Earth divinely
We came to the Earth divinely
So, Man He and She, set your spirit free

I introduce High Priest Kwatamani

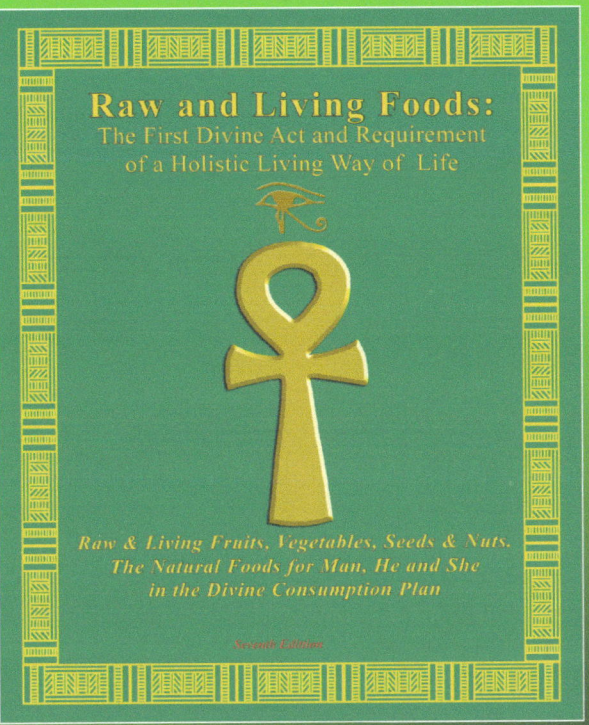

A classic reference source, 1st edition, 1999

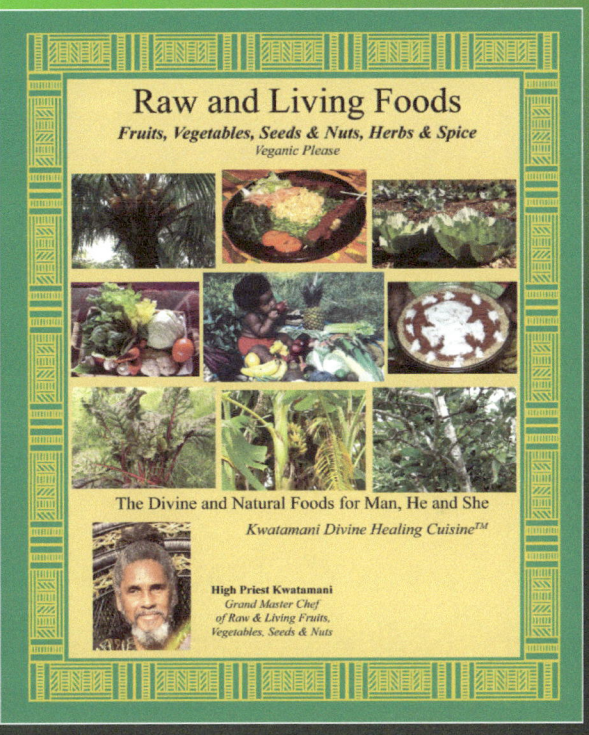

"The subject of raw and living foods is a subject that cannot and must not be taken lightly at this point in time on the planet Earth. The state of being of the malnourished mind of thought is so clouded and so confused and so degenerated and so mutated that, unless there is an urgent and immediate switch—a complete change—to a holistic living lifestyle, the chaos and confusion of this spiritually disconnected and death- oriented mind of thought will completely annihilate the last vestige of the divine mental, physical and spiritual life force of all of those who participate in the consumption of dead and devitalized foods." page, 9.

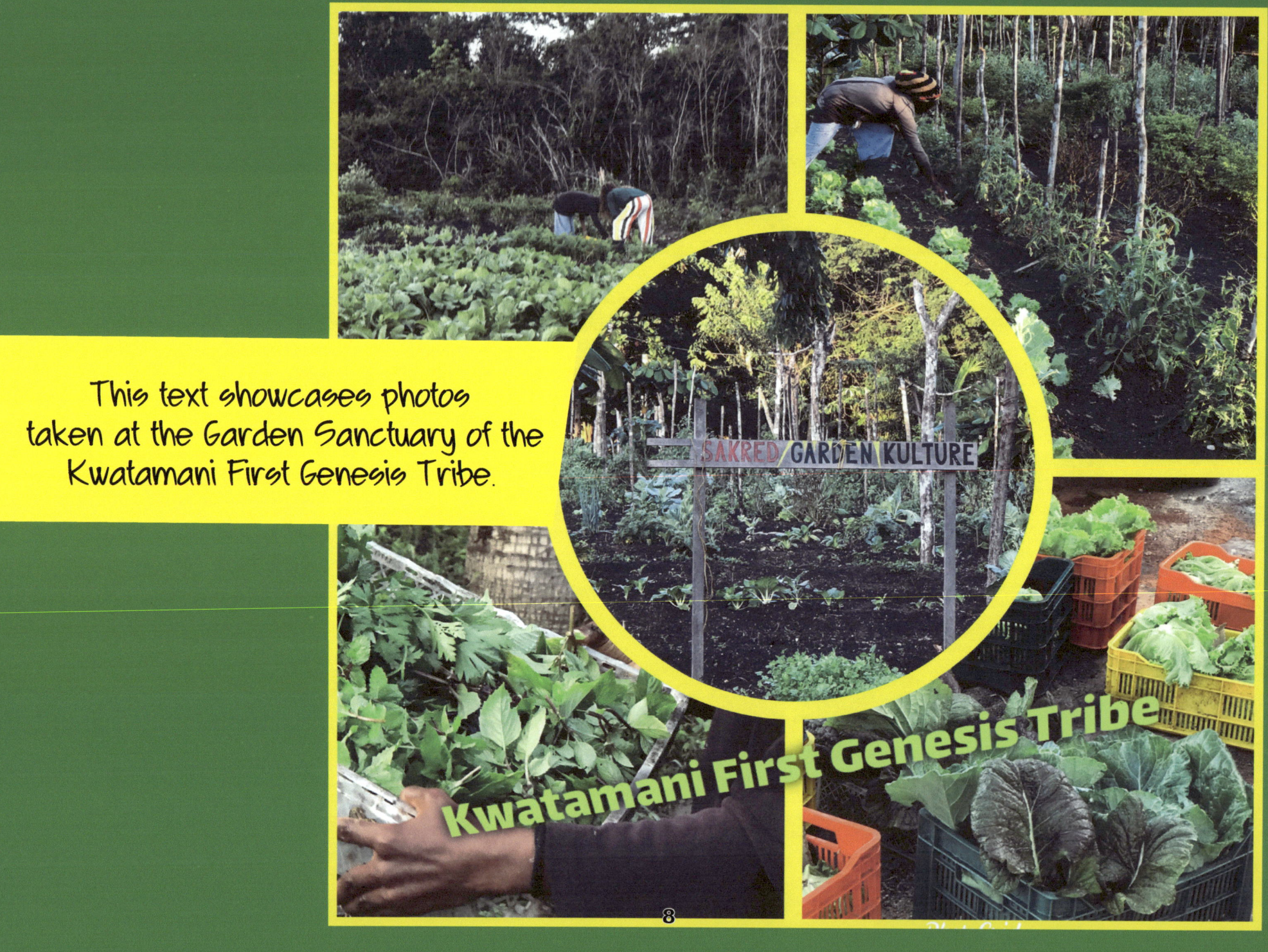

INTRODUCTION: LET FOOD BE YOUR MEDICINE

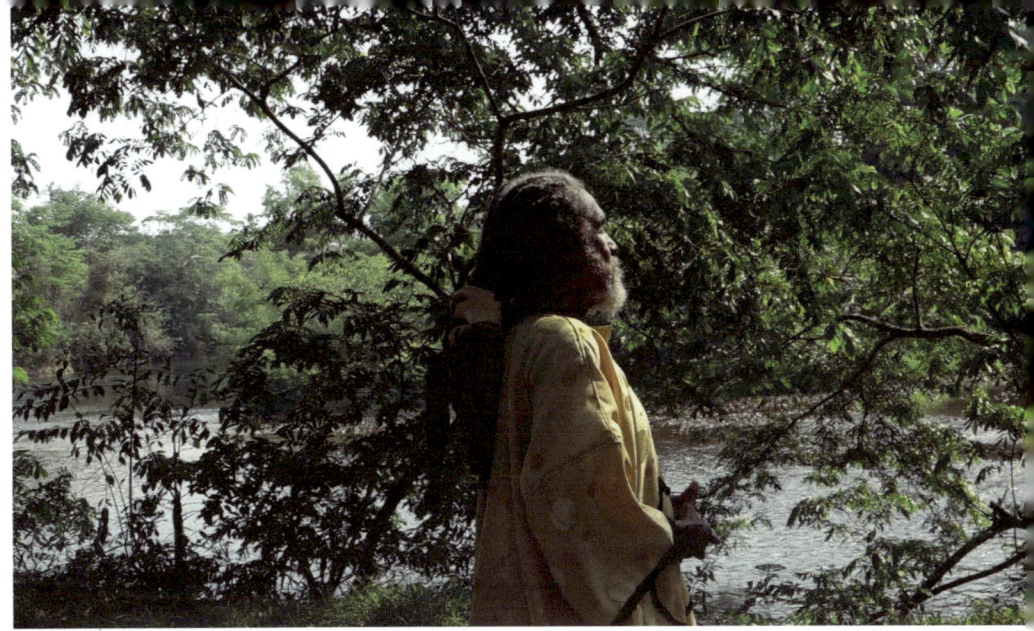

High Priest Kwatamani, Kemetic Naga Priesthood
Sacred Ancestral Temple of Kwa-Ta-Man-I

"Let food be your medicine…" A healing principle historically forwarded by Imhotep, the Kemetic High Priest and healer of ancient Egypt/Kemet. Ancient Egyptians — not ancient Greeks — founded the practice of medicine, according to a study that pushes back the origins at least a thousand years.

Scientists examining documents dating back 3,500 years ago, say they have found proof that the origins of modern medicine did not begin with Hippocrates (460BC - 370BC) and the Greeks, but rather began in ancient Egypt with the likes of Imhotep (2667BC - 2648BC), who designed the pyramids of Saqqara and who was elevated to become honored as the god of healing. The research team from the KNH Centre for Biomedical Egyptology at the University of Manchester discovered the evidence in medical papyri written in 1,500 BC — some 1,000 years before Hippocrates was born.

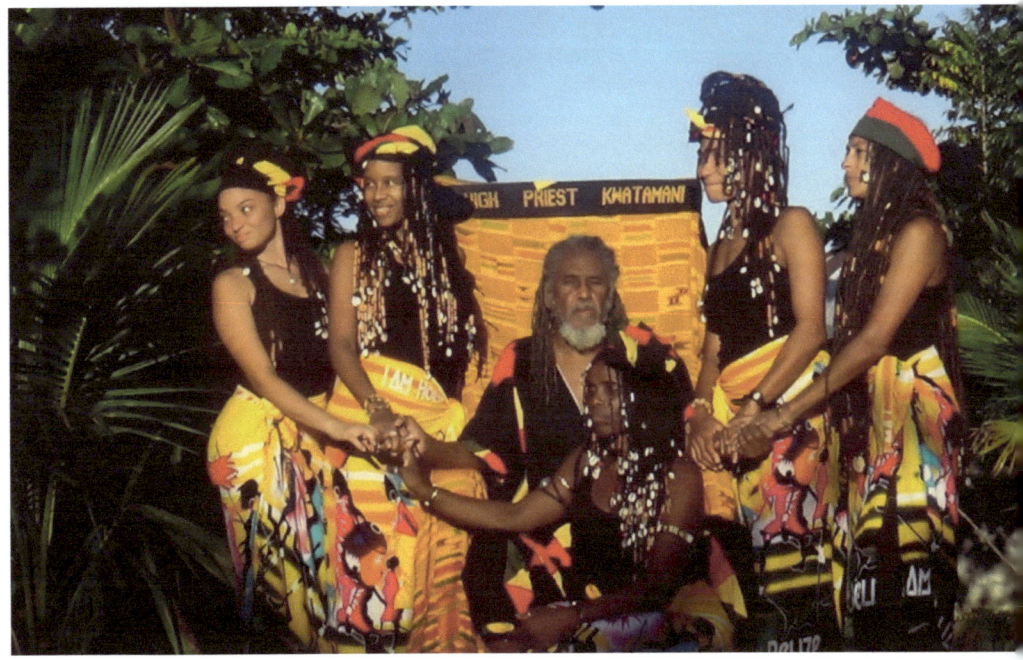

High Priest Kwatamani and the Kwatamani Royal Sisterhood
Kwatamani First Genesis Tribe

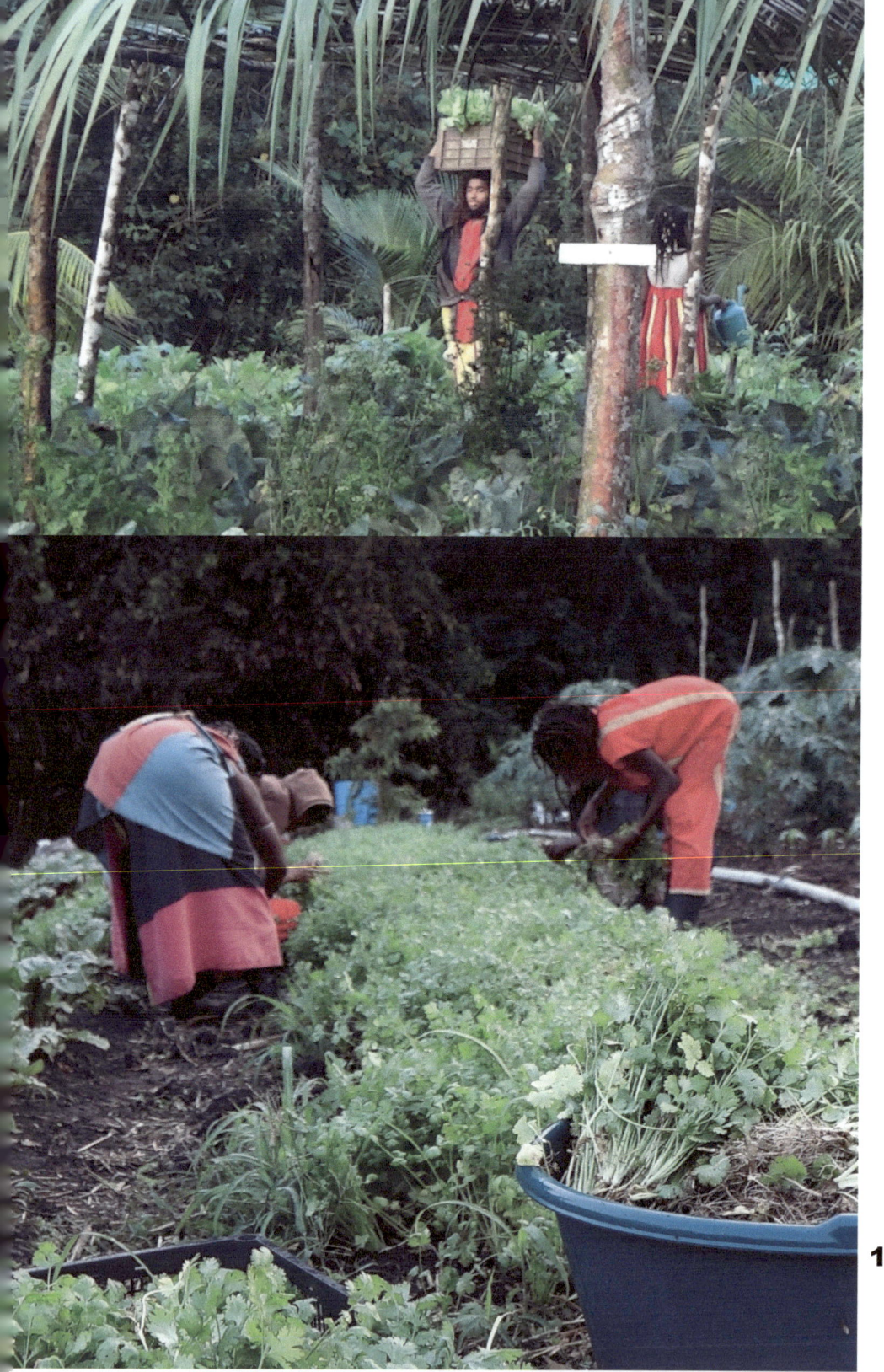

Let's pause for a moment to provide greater clarity during this journey through the sacred ancestral sanctuary of the Kwatamani First Genesis Tribe's Garden of Holistic Living Eating. Here is another quote that stems from the Kemetic Naga priesthood, a quote that has been written, adopted, and spoken, but very seldom followed, by those who never actually knew that within a holistic living way of life, divine actions speak louder than words.

Genesis 1:29 "Behold, I have given you every herb-bearing seed, which is upon the face of the earth and every tree that has seed-yielding fruit – to you it shall be for food."

"Out of the black wholeness of all that we be of supreme ancestral masculine and feminine energy came the divine union of Man, He and She, natural and innate consumers of the fruit of the tree, a divine necessity to forward the multiplication of divinity into divine social economic family community, our holistic living reality. Spoken to be re-awoken."

High Priest Kwatamani
Seeds of the Awoke musical album.

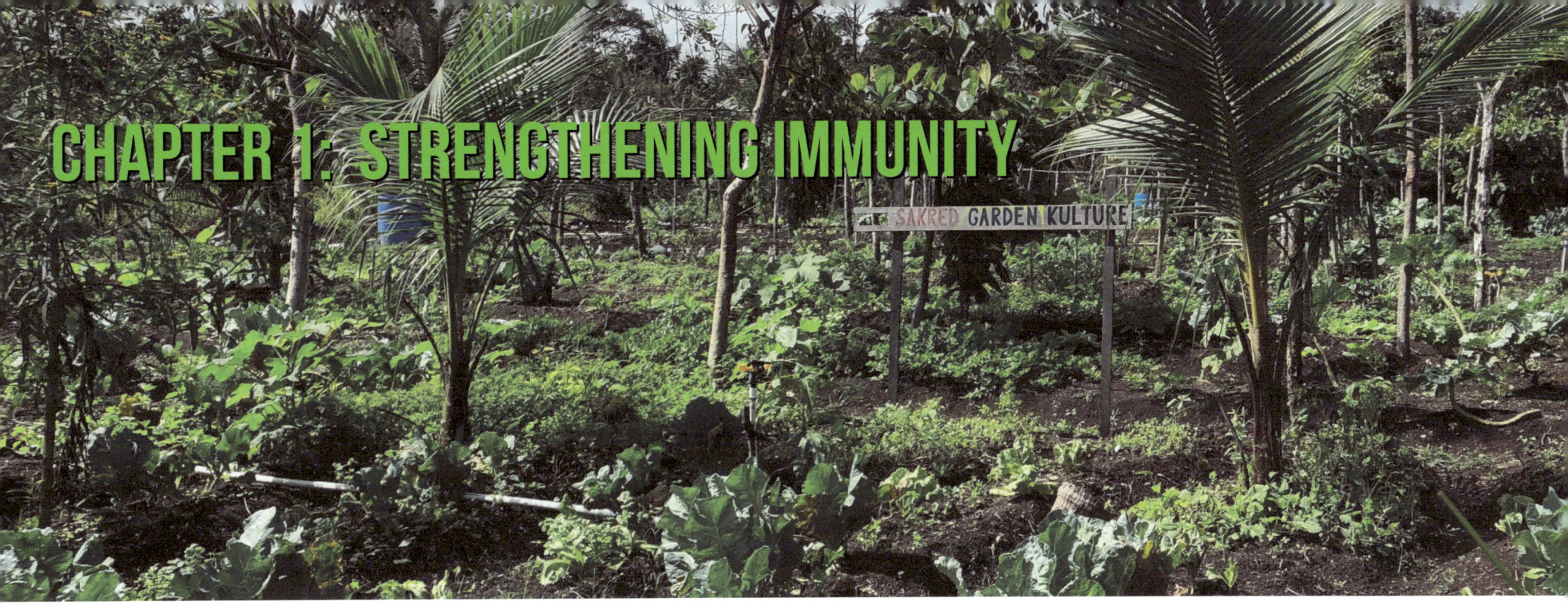

CHAPTER 1: STRENGTHENING IMMUNITY

Holistic Living Survival

What became clear to all of humanity during this prophetic third cycle of nine that began in 2018 and ends in 2027 is that strengthening our immune defense system is key to survival. We are talking about about that magnificent species identified as Man, He and She. In other words, we are talking about the holistic living survival of humanity that goes far beyond the divisions of race, sex or religion. This text focuses on providing information regarding consumption of the kind and type of foods that will not only support the healing factors of humanity but also help to strengthen the immune defense system so as to maintain a state of wholesome health and well-being. Optimum nutrition is definitely a safe, effective and time-proven method of protecting, securing and enhancing one's mental, physical and spiritual state of being. Optimum fuel supports strong and vibrant functioning – optimum performance.

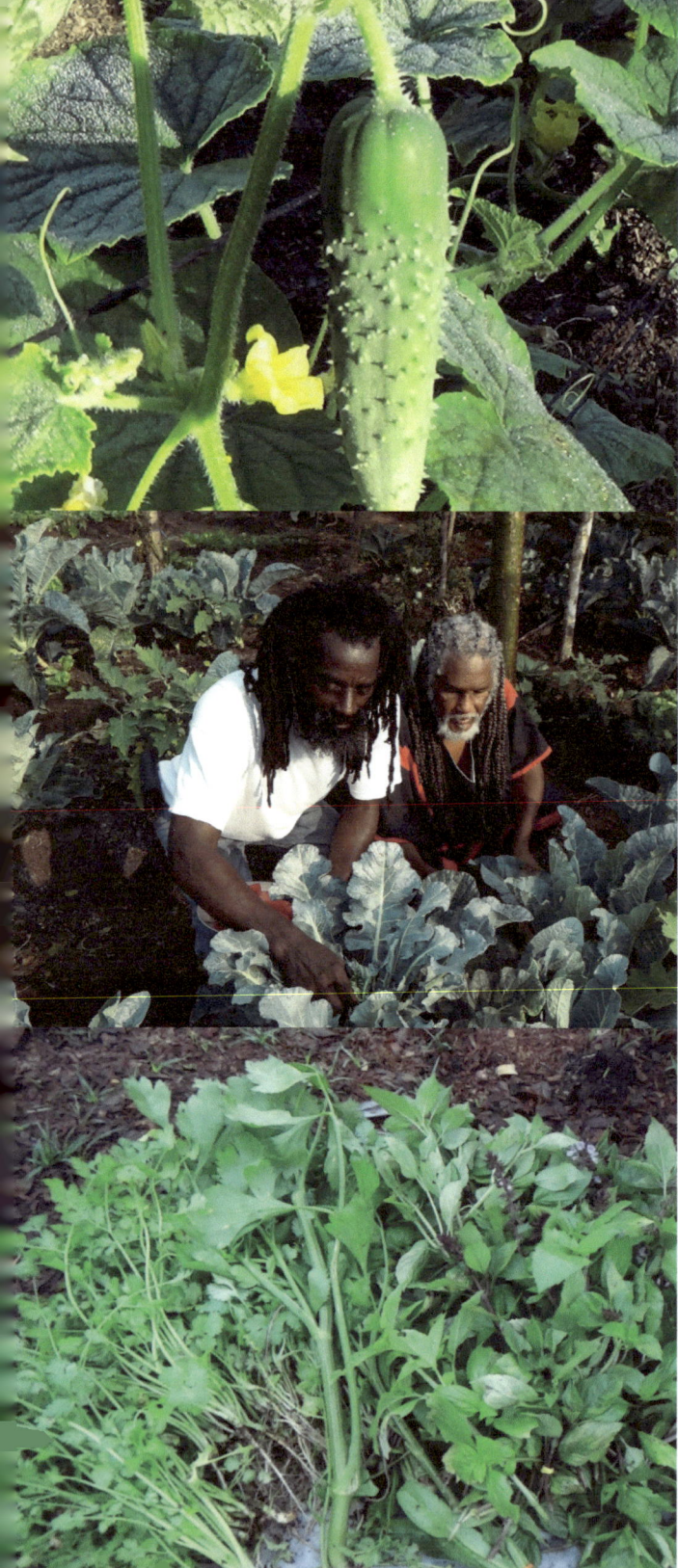

The ancient Kemetic Naga Priesthood teachings include simple principles, such as: You are what you eat. This universal principle defines every holistic living system within the Circle of Life. What you put in is what will come out, and what you put out will come back to you again, multiplied.

Lack of fuel, depleted fuel and/or toxic fuel will cause any living system to stop working properly and eventually breakdown. Breakdown is seen as signs and symptoms of disorder, disease and destructive behaviors that have one final conclusion. Your body, the larger social body, and the collective body of humanity, require fuel.

After observing the nutritional patterns under Western influence for well over half a century, what has become clear to the I in I, is that consuming a mediocre diet has become acceptable and even encouraged. And the accepted and encouraged diet has been shown to produce a lower and lesser energy of fuel that does deplete rather than enhance the immune defense system of the body.

Life-Sustaining Fueling Source

Sacred ancestral wisdom shows us that consuming from any fueling source that is disconnected from the Supreme Circle of Life seriously

CHAPTER 1: STRENGTHENING IMMUNITY

threatens the mental, physical and/or spiritual health and well-being of the individual.

As can be witnessed, many individuals consume without regard for the adverse effects upon their own body, the larger social body of humanity, Mother Earth or any life matters thereof. Yes, the nature of energy that one consumes can disconnect one from the Supreme Circle of Life, i.e. the circle of divine social-economic family-community order. Disconnection from a life-sustaining fueling source can cause sickness, disease and disorder as the truth and consequence of unhealthy, unwholesome consumption. As one disconnects from the Supreme Circle of Life, one automatically connects to the vicious circle that fuels the divisive nature of self-asserted individualism, and the conflict, confusion and chaos that it manifests. The vicious circle breeds the survival-of-the-fittest mentality. A vicious circle controlled by warlords, conquerors,

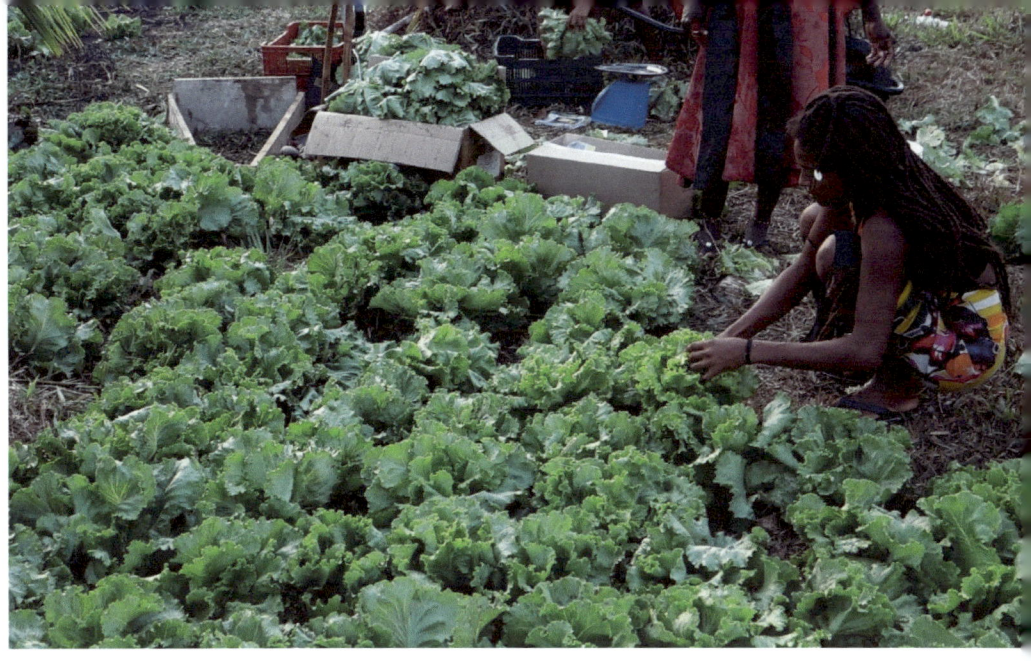

hunters, and herders, a vicious circle that is hazardous to the health of those targeted for invasion, conquest, enslavement, and destruction. Unfortunately, the survival-of-the-fittest mentality dominates, controls and projects superiority as the ruling force of our planet today. That is to say, superior blood spillers, killers and enforcers of an enslaving mindset that perpetuates greed and lust while polluting and violating the body of Mother Earth. This same mentality breeds disregard and disrespect for the sacred ancestral feminine nature that birthed humanity, i.e. Mother Nature and the feminine

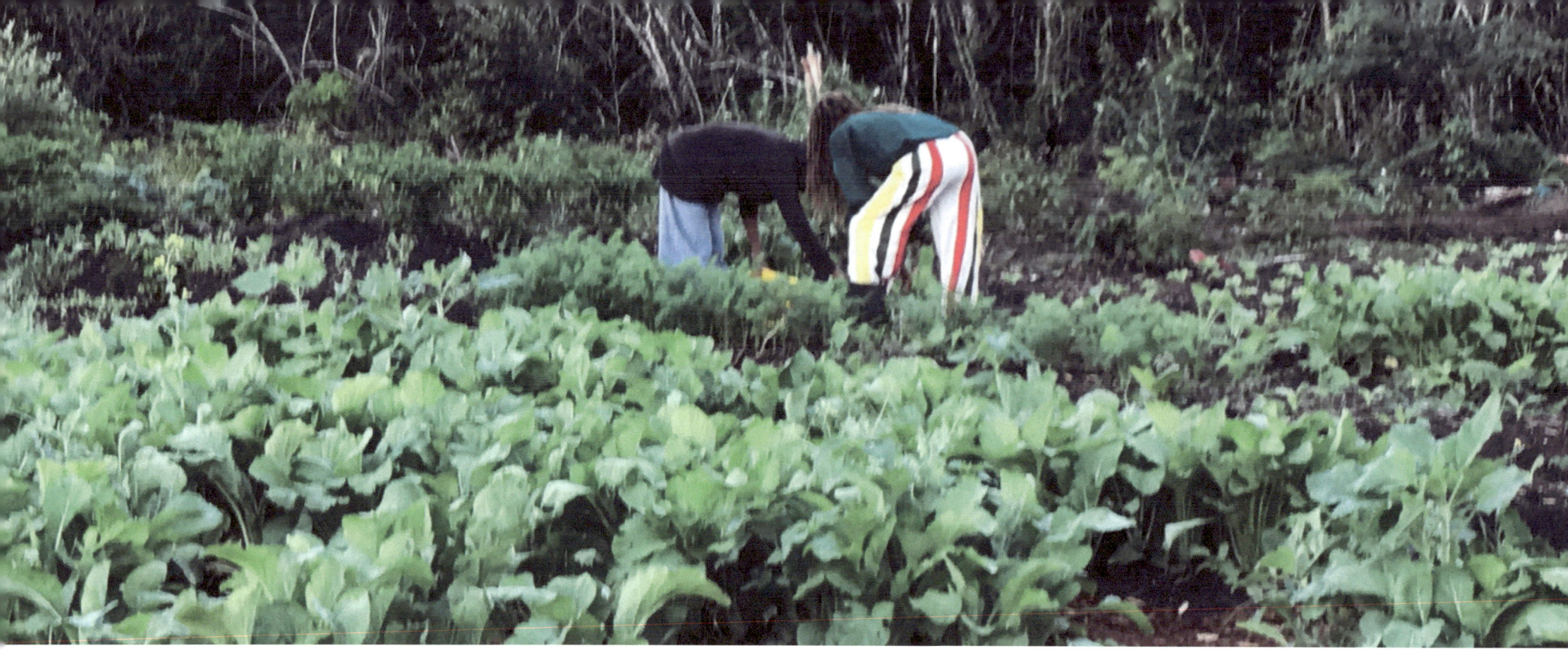

She. Thus, disregard and disrespect were seeded, bred and fed into the consciousness of so many among humanity. This consciousness spreads a virus-like plague of conflict, confusion and chaotic sickness, disease and disorder as a way of life. We are talking about an unhealthy way of life that actually undermines the natural immune defense system's ability to protect and safeguard one's mental, physical and spiritual state of being. That's right, what we are saying is that the natural and innate order of earth, wind, rain and sun is requiring Man, He and She, to submit to a holistic earth-solar-conscious way of life or die. Submit or die from the virus-like plague of dead, devitalized and depleted energy that is infecting all who consume of it. Right now we are going to focus on the immune system, but remember that no living cell or organ

CHAPTER 1: STRENGTHENING IMMUNITY

functions in isolation within your body. Your body is a collective, a holistic living system that includes all parts working together. This is why a holistic living way of life forwards the whole life presence of each and every Man, He and She, as members of the collective body of humanity. We refer to the state of health and wholesome well-being as the divine order of universal law. Health is the holistic living wealth of humanity.

Why Nutrition is Key

With all due honor to the Kemetic Naga Priesthood, the I in I state again that you are what you eat. If you consume of dead, devitalized and depleted energy, you will produce a dead, devitalized and depleted consciousness. And a dead, devitalized and depleted state of consciousness will corrupt the health of your body temple, and will ultimately cause the corruption of the essence of your existence, that is, your soul.

Before we go any further, we say that this text is for all who sincerely seek whole life healing, regardless of the divisive perceptions and profiles of race, creed, color, sex or national origin. Thus, healing one's soul, that is to say, spiritual healing, has everything to do with the nature of energy you consume, mentally and physically. That's right, this text is written to resurrect the sacred ancestral soul of humanity... So, let's do it in the most supreme spirit of love.

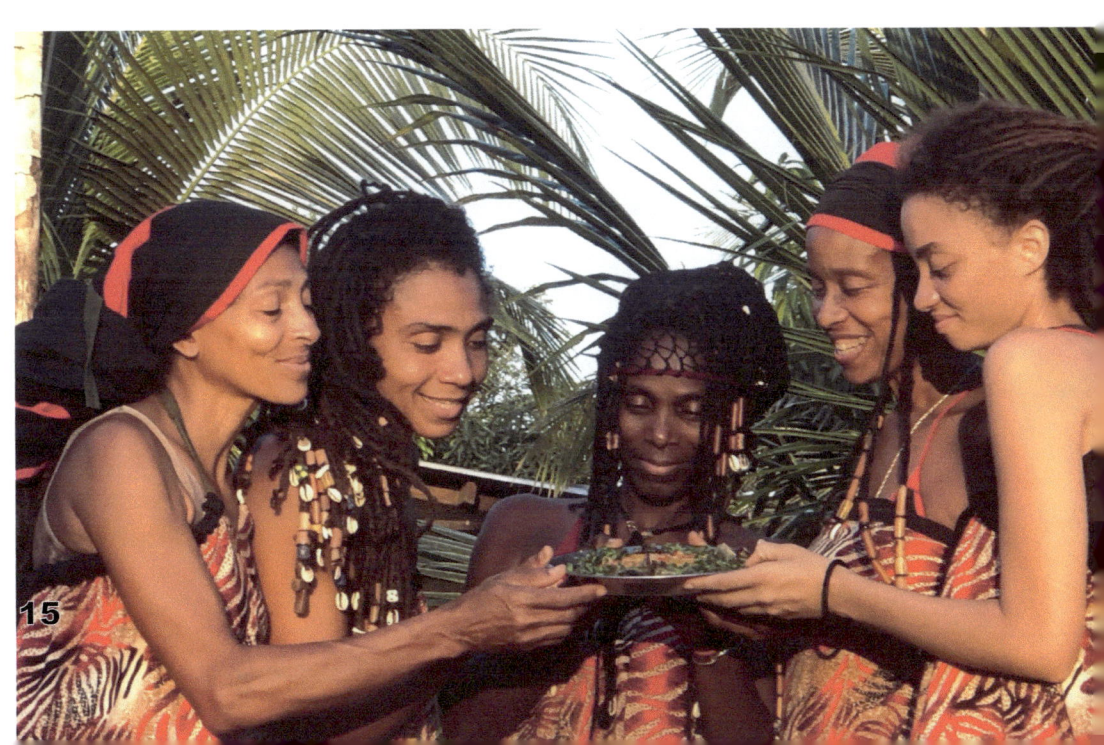

CODE GREEN: HIDDEN POWERS OF THE GARDEN TARGETING THE IMMUNE SYSTEM

Viruses, Bacteria, Protozoa & Fungi

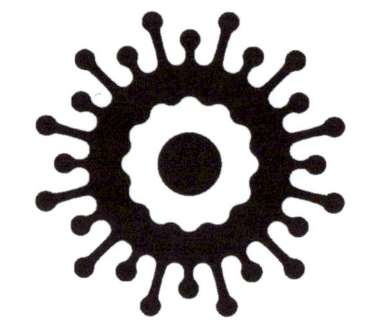
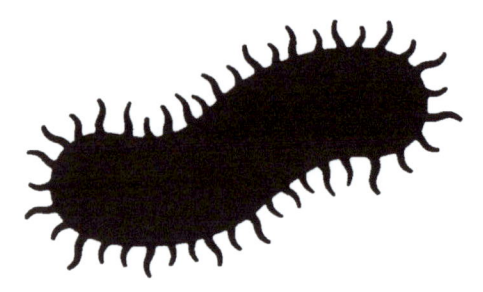

Before one can get a solution to any problem, one must comprehend the nature of the problem. The problem is that sickness, disease and disorder occurs because of nutrient deficiencies and/or foreign substances invading the body. When the body is invaded by harmful foreign substances such as bacteria, viruses, parasites and toxins, the first response is for the immune system to do its job.

Viruses are microscopic parasites, generally much smaller than bacteria. They lack the ability to thrive and reproduce outside of a host body. "The primary role of the virus is to deliver its DNA or RNA gene code into a host cell so that it can be expressed by the host cell," according to Medical Microbiology. And one then becomes infected.

Bacteria are microscopic living organisms, usually one-celled. They can be beneficial or harmful.

Protozoa are one-celled organisms that are known to cause diseases such as malaria.

Fungi are spore-producing organisms that feed on organic matter. Fungi include molds, mildew, yeast, and mushrooms.

Harmful invading substances are called pathogens

Antibodies are specialized proteins in the immune system that protect the body against infection by pathogens which cause disease.

This protection is called immunity.

Antibodies
BUILDING DEFENSE

- Antibodies are proteins produced by the immune system.

- Antibodies defend against specific foreign substances, such as bacteria, viruses, fungi, parasites, toxins etc.

- Antibodies neutralize toxins (poisonous or damaging substances) produced by different organisms

- Antibodies activate a group of proteins that help eliminate bacteria, viruses and infected cells

Immune System Fundamentals

Strong defense and protection from harmful invading forces is essential during these times of increased contamination in the environment. The immune system protects the body against infection and disease. It is known to be an integrated system of cells, tissues and organs with specialized roles in defending against foreign substances and pathogenic microorganisms, including bacteria, viruses and fungi.

▶ The front-line defense in our bodies provides physical barriers and chemical barriers, such as the skin, mucus, stomach acids, tears, etc., and also biological barriers such as microflora in the intestines.

▶ The second line of defense is immune responses that can produce fever and inflammation.

▶ The third line is immune responses that produce defense cells that help neutralize, eliminate and destroy harmful invasive substances.

When all three lines of defense fail, the individual is said to get sick and is subject to disease.

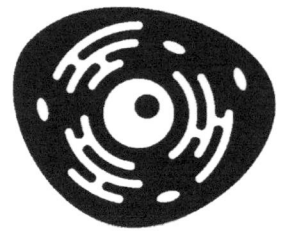 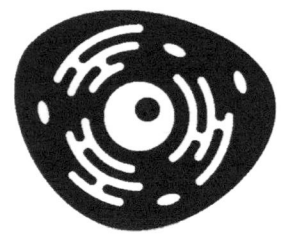 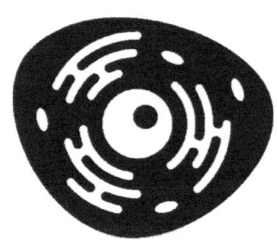

Cells of the immune system originate in the bone marrow and circulate to the peripheral tissues in the blood and the lymph. Organs of the immune system include the thymus, spleen and lymph nodes. Research indicates that the immune system is broadly divided into two major parts: the innate immunity and adaptive immunity. Research also shows that the innate system includes a biochemical network of more than 30 proteins in the blood plasma as well as immune defense cells that have an immediate response to invading pathogens.

The adaptive system is said to take several days or weeks to fully develop, including the immune memory. Immune memory means that immune response upon a second exposure to the same pathogen are faster and stronger because the pathogen has been identified and remembered.

There are front-line defenders in the form of colorless blood cells that are called white blood cells. Some types of white blood cells break down invading organisms. Other defender cells are known to help the body remember the invasive substances and destroy them. These cells function as the body's security intelligence system – they find their targets and send defenses to lock them down.

The defense cells are triggered to make antibodies which remain present to protect the body against foreign matter that is not of the body. Antibodies work to identify foreign matter, but they need the help of T-cells which function to destroy substances that have been identified as harmful.

(Some T cells are actually called "killer cells.") T-cells also signal other cells in the immune system to defend against harmful substances that threaten the healthy functioning of the body.

CHAPTER 1: STRENGTHENING IMMUNITY

Nutritional Support Is A Must

Healthy eating habits and lifestyle habits aid in boosting the body's natural defenses. Don't forget to drink plenty of water. Water helps your body produce lymph, which carries white blood cells and other immune system cells.

> "The healing energies of plant-based consumption are one of the many blessings of the Sacred Garden Culture from which we come. However, many brains have been programmed to think, reason, and act within the hunting-and-herding consumption patterns of cooked foods and animal flesh while overdosing on salt, sugar, and grease. The nutritional needs of the brain have been sacrificed to the lusting appetites of the Self-asserting will that has no care for the body or the brain, except as a tool to be used to satisfy the Deified Self."

The Ausarian Sacred Ancestral Temple of KRIST (KRIST text), p.146

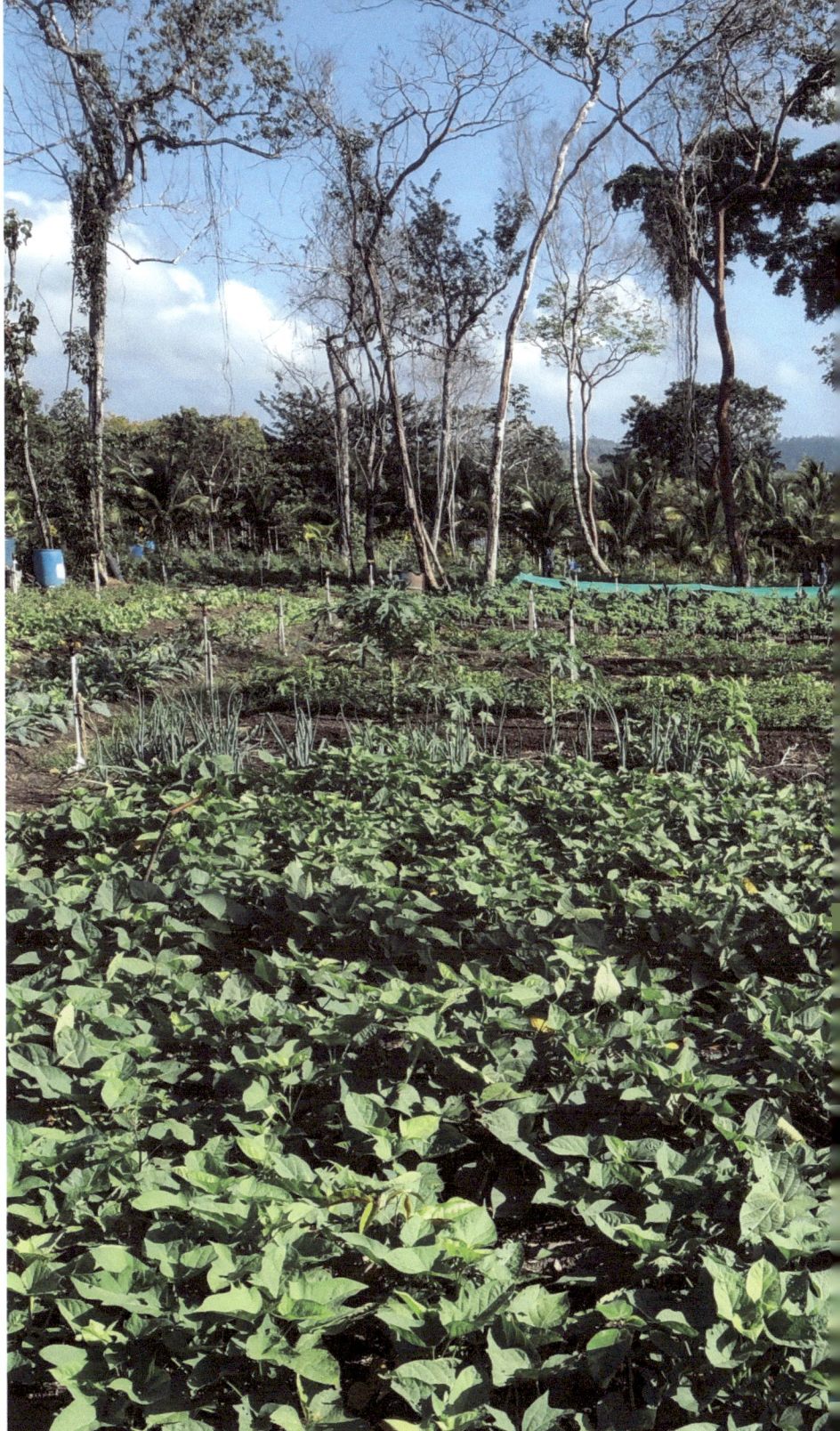

Eat more fruits and vegetables to greatly increase antibody response.

20

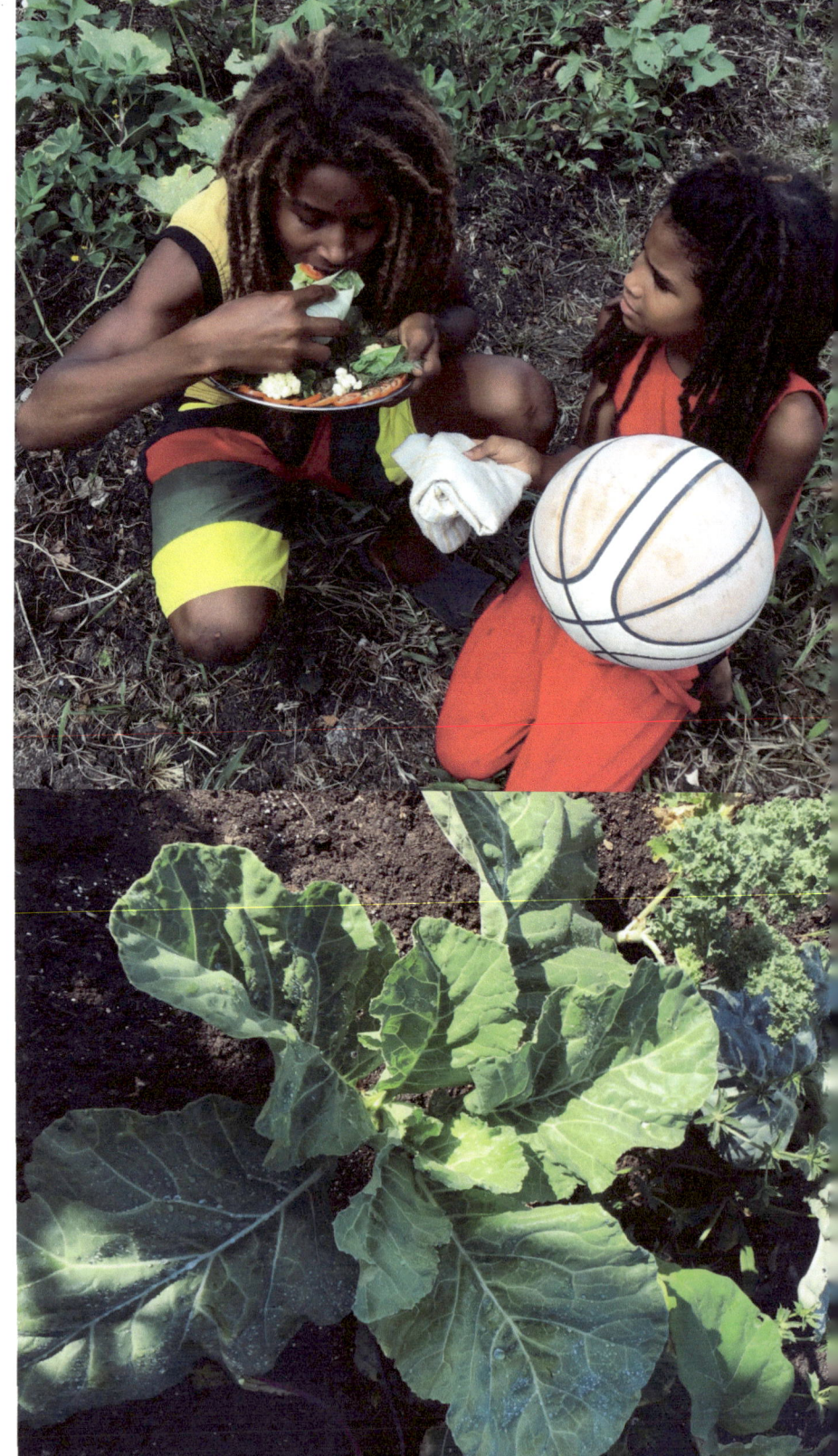

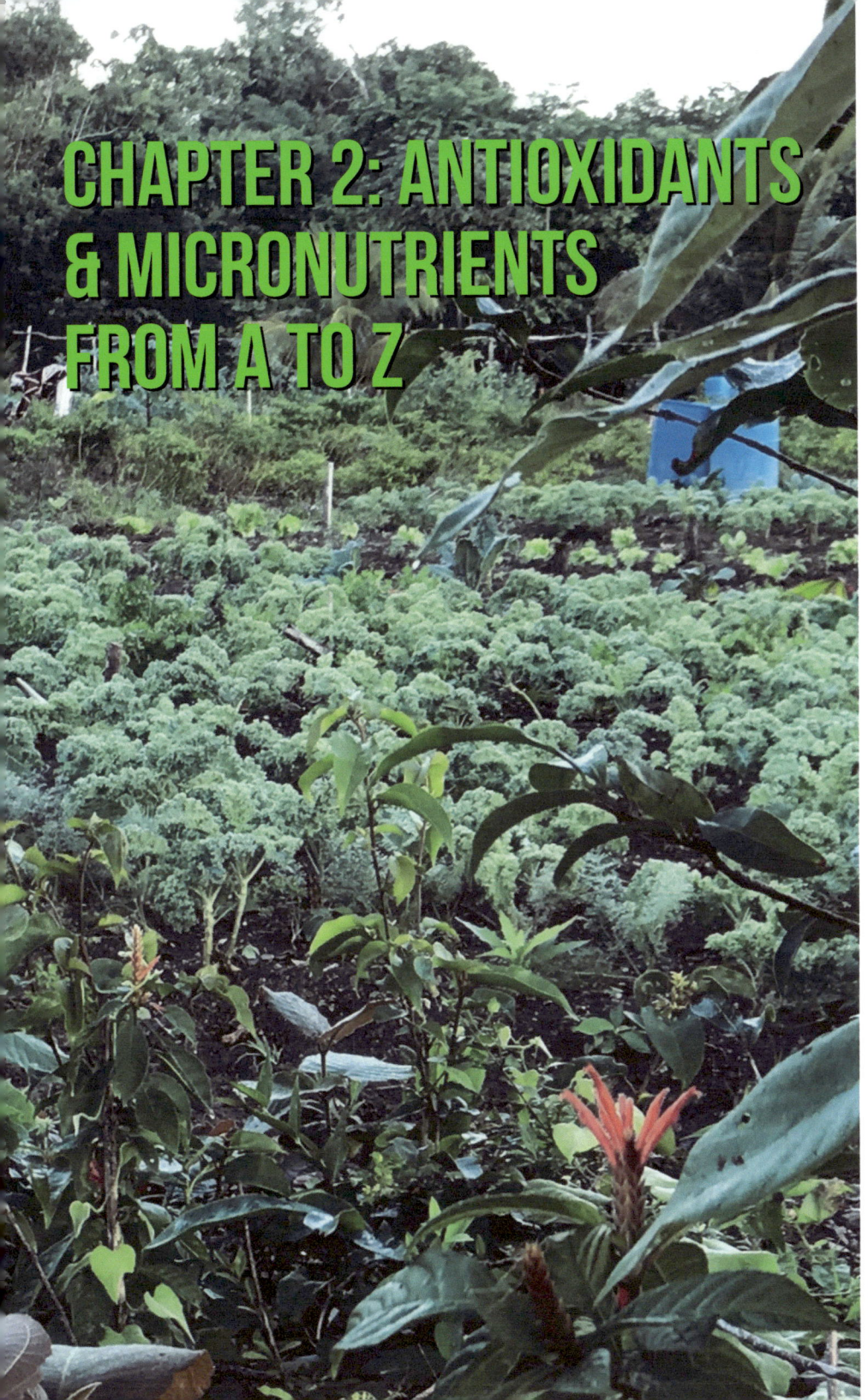

CHAPTER 2: ANTIOXIDANTS & MICRONUTRIENTS FROM A TO Z

The first line of defense to protect and maintain a wholesome and healthy state of being begins in the brain, the communication center of the body. The brain processes thoughts and reasoning and signals actions to safeguard one's health. A sense of harmony and balance and the ability to neutralize stress helps to support a positive mental attitude. The brain requires high-level nutrients and lots of oxygen to function. The brain's need for oxygen is more than ten times greater than the need of the rest of the body. Studies show that when oxygen is converted into energy, the process produces unstable molecules called free radicals.

When produced in balanced amounts, free radicals work to rid the body of harmful toxins. However when produced in excessive amounts, these so-called free radicals create chemical reactions that damage healthy cells sometimes faster than the cells can be repaired. Research indicates that free radicals can also impair the functioning of the immune system. We will highlight those well-identified nutrients that are

In simple terms, an antioxidant is a substance that slows or delays specific types of cell damage.

Vitamins A, C and E are among the most noted antioxidants.

These are abundant in many fresh fruits and vegetables.

reported to greatly support efficient functioning of the immune system.

Vitamin A

Vitamin A is very important in supporting the immune system. Vitamin A helps maintain the mucus lining of the respiratory and gastrointestinal tract to protect against infection. This vitamin strengthens the adaptive immune system to help fight invasive viruses and bacteria.

Vitamin A deficiency can lead to muscular degeneration, including degeneration of the muscles of the heart and infections of the ear, nose, mouth and respiratory system. Some foods with high concentrations of vitamin A are carrots, corn off of the cob, sweet potatoes, winter squash, broccoli, lettuce, cabbage, leafy green vegetables like spinach, kale, (sweet) potato greens, collard greens; dandelion, turnip, mustard and beet greens; watercress, parsley, apricots, oranges, cantaloupes, mangoes, papaya, peaches, prunes, watermelon, pecans and peppers. *Raw and Living Foods, p. 44.*

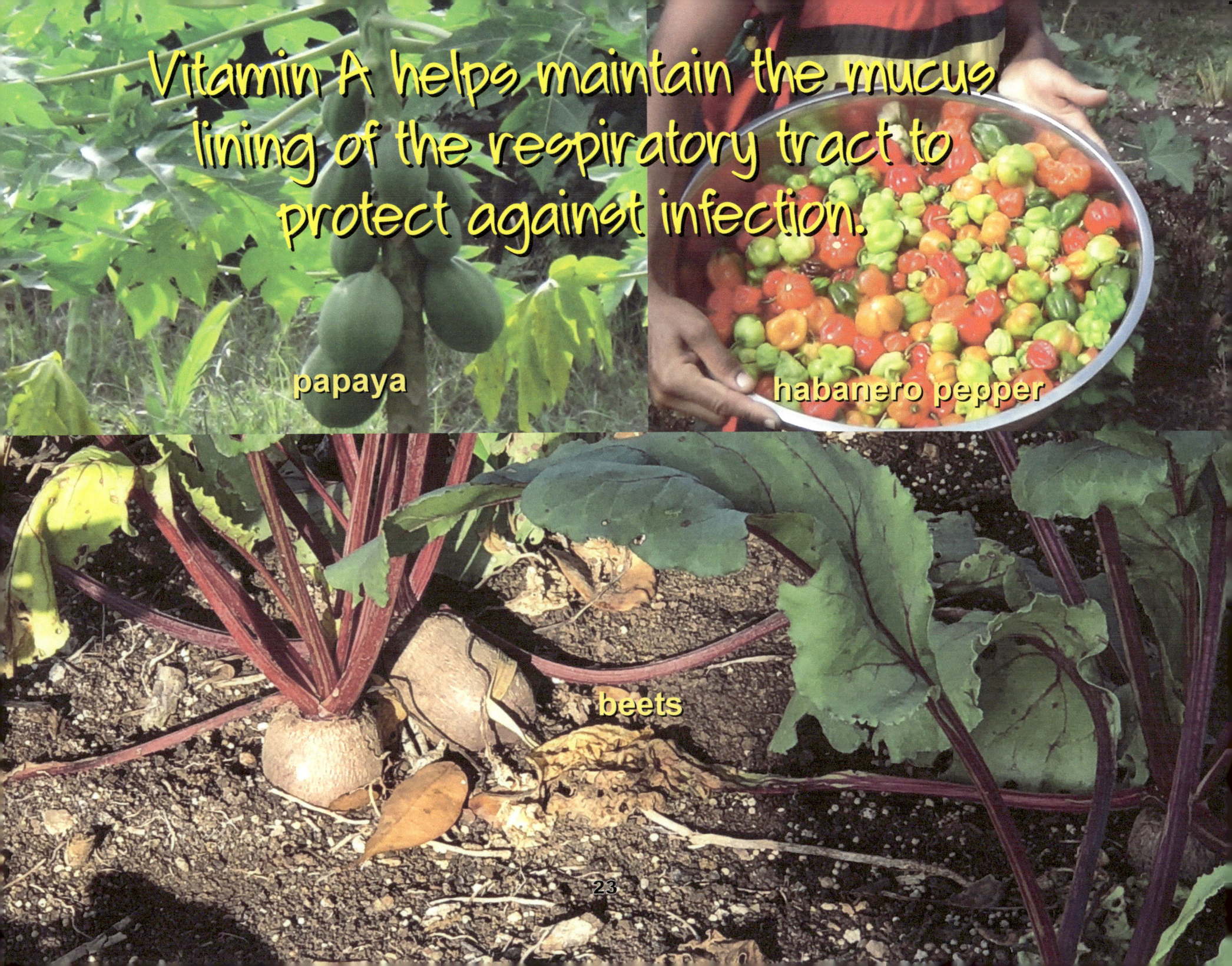

Special Focus

NUTRITIONAL PROTECTION

- Vitamin A (Beta Carotene)
- Vitamin B Complex
- Vitamin C
- Vitamin D
- Vitamin E
- Zinc

CODE GREEN: HIDDEN POWERS OF THE GARDEN TARGETING THE IMMUNE SYSTEM

Plants provide a most potent source of Vitamin A in the form carotenoids which are the pigments that give plants their green color and some fruits and vegetables their red or orange color. For instance, sweet potatoes are far superior than the run-of-the-mill white potato. The orange variety contains beta carotene, which makes them filled with robust antioxidant, antiviral, and anticancer abilities. They're also full of fiber, and the vitamin E they contain is healthy for the skin.

Beets are high in vitamins A and C, calcium, iron, potassium and sodium. They also contain significant amounts of folic acid, vitamin B_6, choline, chromium, fluorine, magnesium, manganese, potassium, phosphorus, silicon and sulfur. Beets are excellent blood-builders, building the red corpuscles. The beet is also a powerful blood and liver cleanser.

CHAPTER 2: ANTIOXIDANTS & MICRONUTRIENTS FROM A TO Z

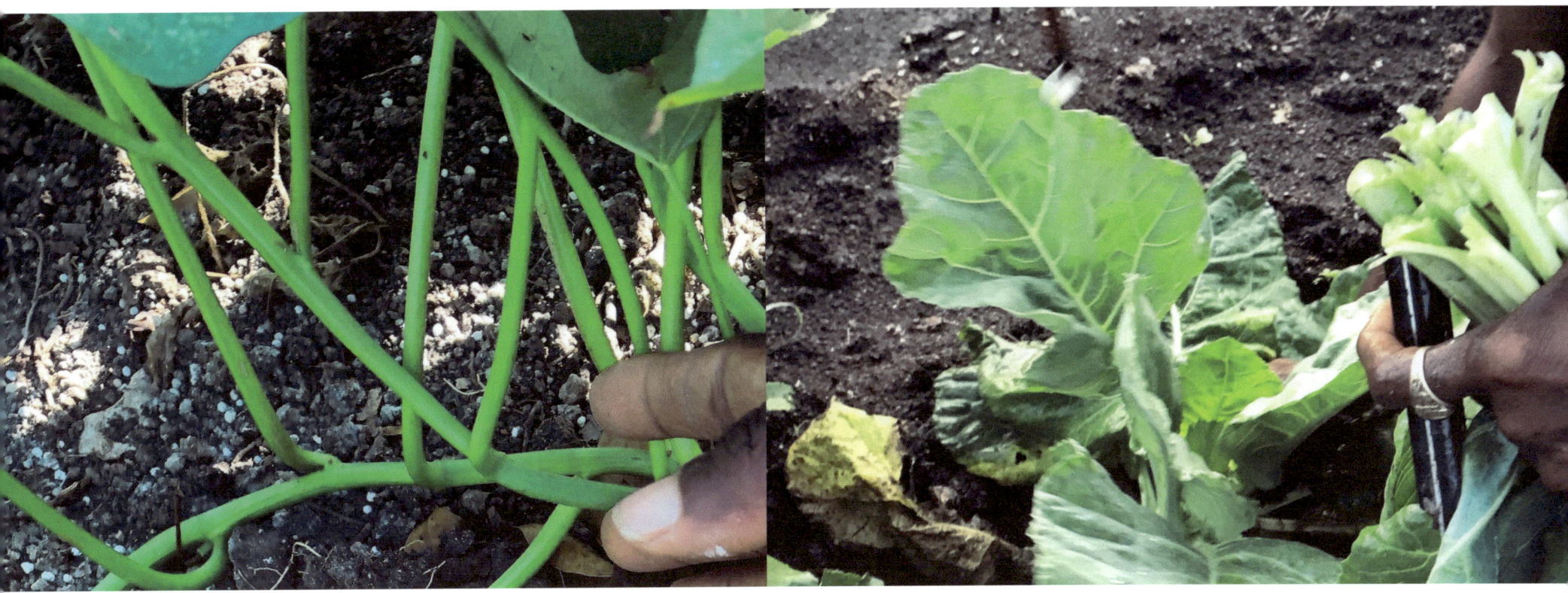

Vitamin B

Vitamin B refers to not one, but eight different vitamins. All B vitamins play a role in converting food into energy in the body.

Vitamin B_6 is required for the synthesis and metabolism of amino acids – the building blocks of proteins like antibodies and other defense proteins of the immune system. In particular, there is evidence that folic acid (vitamin B_9) and cobalamin (vitamin B_{12}) play a crucial role in the healthy balance of the immune system. Inadequate levels of B_9 and B_{12} can drastically alter immune responses by affecting the production of nucleic acid and protein synthesis, inhibiting the activity of immune cells. Vitamin B_{12} is necessary for proper red blood cell formation, including the proper functioning of the blood-

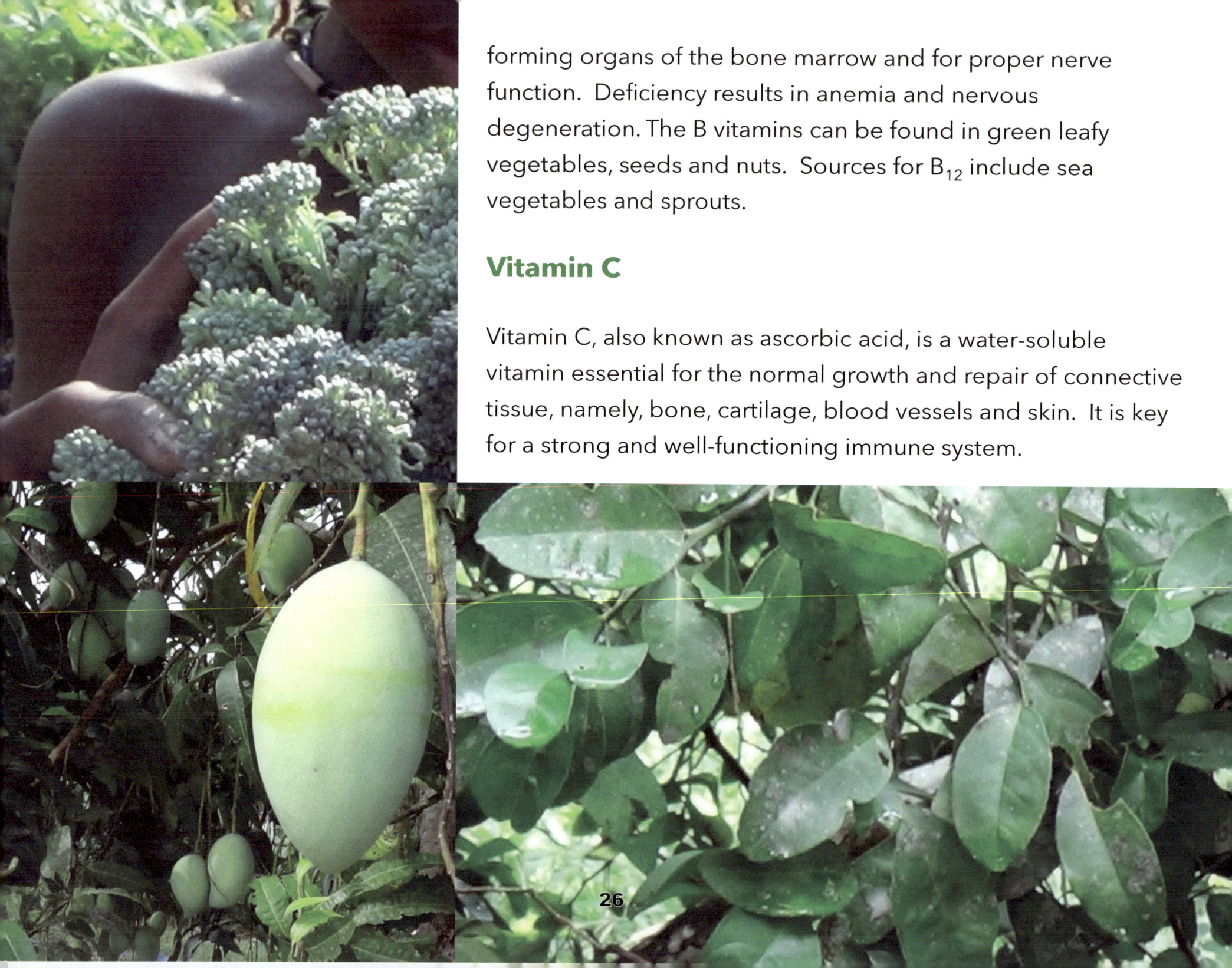

forming organs of the bone marrow and for proper nerve function. Deficiency results in anemia and nervous degeneration. The B vitamins can be found in green leafy vegetables, seeds and nuts. Sources for B_{12} include sea vegetables and sprouts.

Vitamin C

Vitamin C, also known as ascorbic acid, is a water-soluble vitamin essential for the normal growth and repair of connective tissue, namely, bone, cartilage, blood vessels and skin. It is key for a strong and well-functioning immune system.

CHAPTER 2: ANTIOXIDANTS & MICRONUTRIENTS FROM A TO Z

Vitamin C stimulates both the production and function of white blood cells which work to ward off infection. Vitamin C is reported to enhance communication proteins released from white blood cells, thus promoting the immune response. There is some evidence that vitamin C may be particularly helpful in boosting the immune systems of people under major stress.

Studies show that Vitamin C is also necessary for what has been reported as "cellular death", which helps keep the immune system healthy by clearing out old, damaged cells. To increase your vitamin C intake, add more of these fruits and vegetables to your daily meals: red and green bell peppers, oranges, strawberries, broccoli, cauliflower, mangoes, lemons, limes, and many more.

Red bell pepper is bursting with vitamin C, making it a powerful immune builder. If you think citrus fruits have the most vitamin C of any fruit or vegetable, think again. Ounce for ounce, red bell peppers contain twice as much vitamin C as citrus. Cauliflower, also noted as providing Vitamin C, is noted to be a good blood purifier.

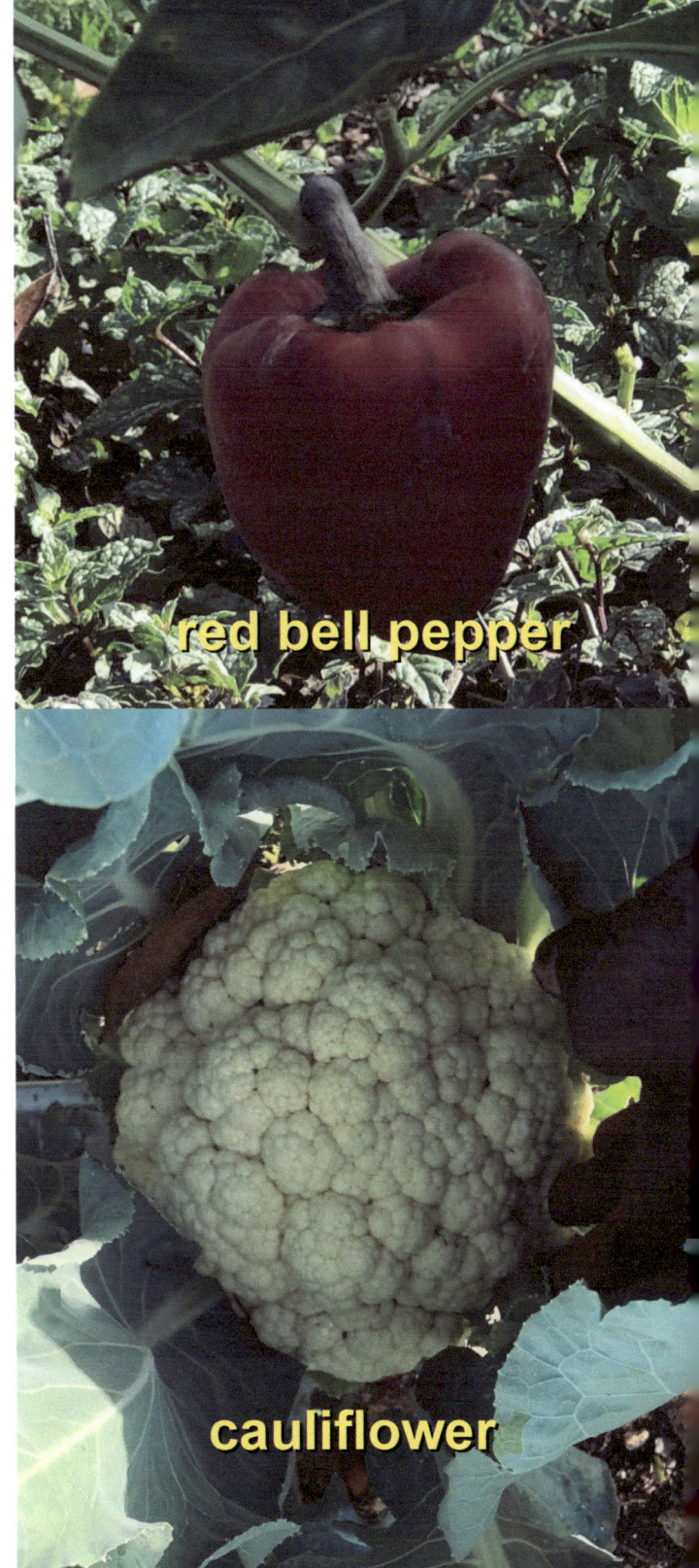
red bell pepper

cauliflower

CODE GREEN: HIDDEN POWERS OF THE GARDEN TARGETING THE IMMUNE SYSTEM

Vitamin D

We of the Kwatamani First Genesis Tribe honor the three basic needs of life as essential: food, sunshine and tender, loving care. We call vitamin D the sunshine vitamin. Vitamin D is a fat soluble nutrient essential to the health and functioning of your immune system. Vitamin D helps to regulate the immune system to quickly identify and destroy pathogens that enter the body. It has been noted that low vitamin D levels are associated with an increased risk of upper respiratory tract infections, including influenza and allergic asthma. Your body synthesizes vitamin D when exposed to sunlight.

Vitamin E

Research suggests maintaining ample levels of vitamin E is crucial for maintaining a healthy immune system, especially among older people.

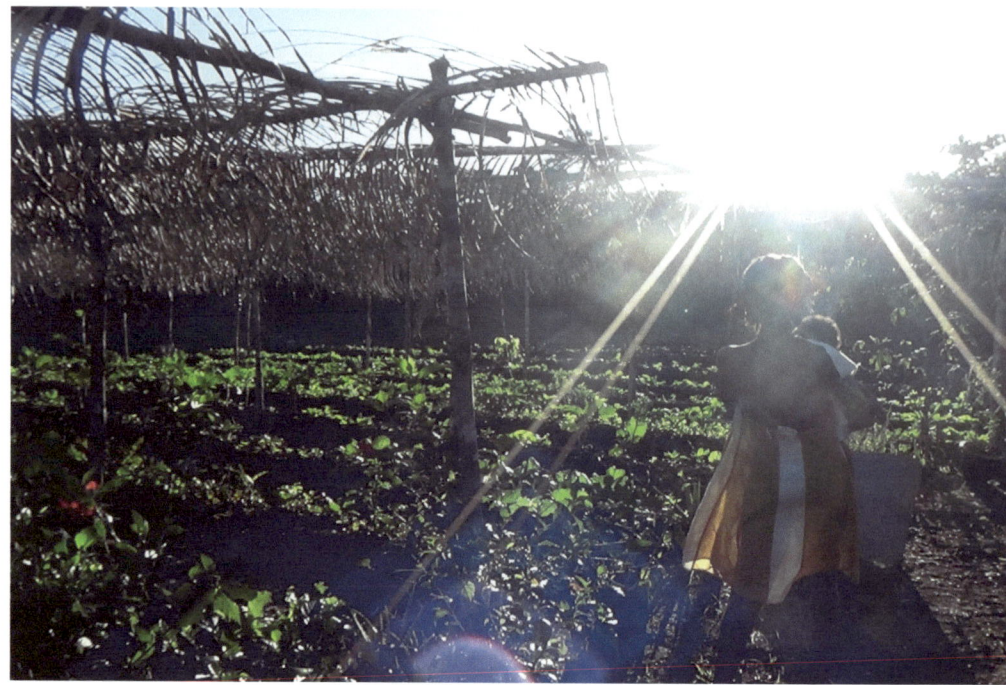

Vitamin D, the sunshine vitamin

Vitamin E is a fat-soluble vitamin, meaning it requires the presence of fat to be absorbed properly. Nuts, such as almonds, are packed with vitamin E and also have healthy fats. Studies show that vitamin E is found in higher concentration in immune cells compared to other cells in the blood. Vitamin E has been shown to enhance the T-cell immune response.

CHAPTER 2: ANTIOXIDANTS & MICRONUTRIENTS FROM A TO Z

Vitamin E is necessary for maintenance of normal red blood cells, proper functioning of the reproductive organs and the metabolization of fats. It aids in proper immune function and helps to prevent blood clots and heart disease.

Deficiency can result in infertility, deterioration of the nervous system, nervousness, irritability, headaches and fatigue; slow growth and defective development of the reproductive cells; and, in women, habitual miscarriage, absence of menstruation, late maturing and infrequent ovulation.

Vitamin E is found in plant oils, whole grains like barley, rye and wheat; asparagus, broccoli, cabbage, corn off the cob, parsnips, sprouts, lettuce, leafy green vegetables, apples, strawberries, cherries, sunflower seeds, almonds, walnuts, peanuts and other nuts.

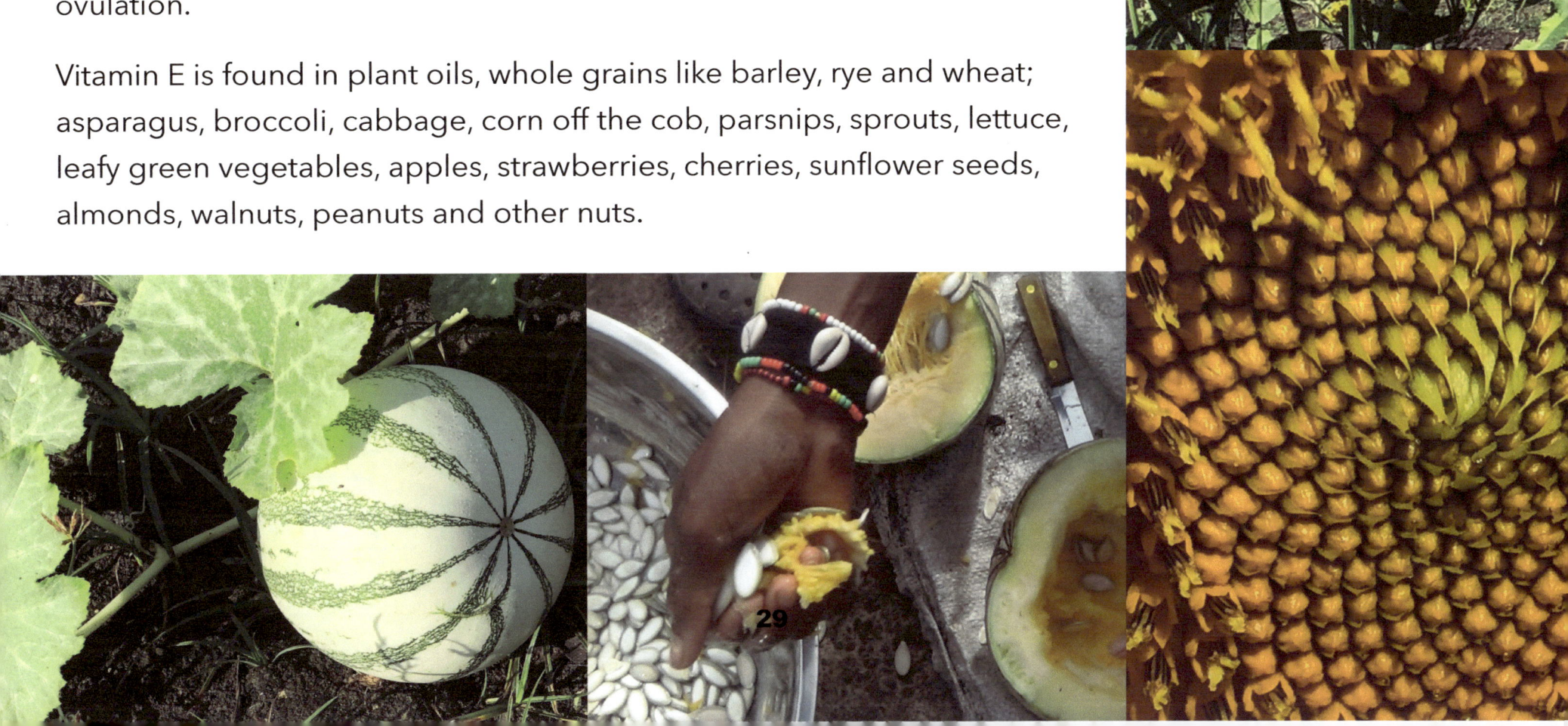

CODE GREEN: HIDDEN POWERS OF THE GARDEN
TARGETING THE IMMUNE SYSTEM

Sesame seeds are a good source of nutrients that are important for immune system function, including zinc, selenium, copper, iron, B_6 and vitamin E. "So, let's forward with sesame seeds, pumpkin seeds, and sunflower seeds, which contain the regenerating energies that reproduce new life. Sesame seeds are very high in minerals such as calcium, magnesium, manganese, copper and iron, and black sesame seeds are especially potent. The I in I have observed over the years that sesame seeds strengthen the reproductive system of both males and females, providing both extra energy and improved stamina.

Sprouting sesame seeds makes them easier to ingest. Seeds and nuts have nutrient factors that help produce nitric oxide in t he body, which relaxes the blood vessels and increases blood flow". *KRIST text, p. 236*

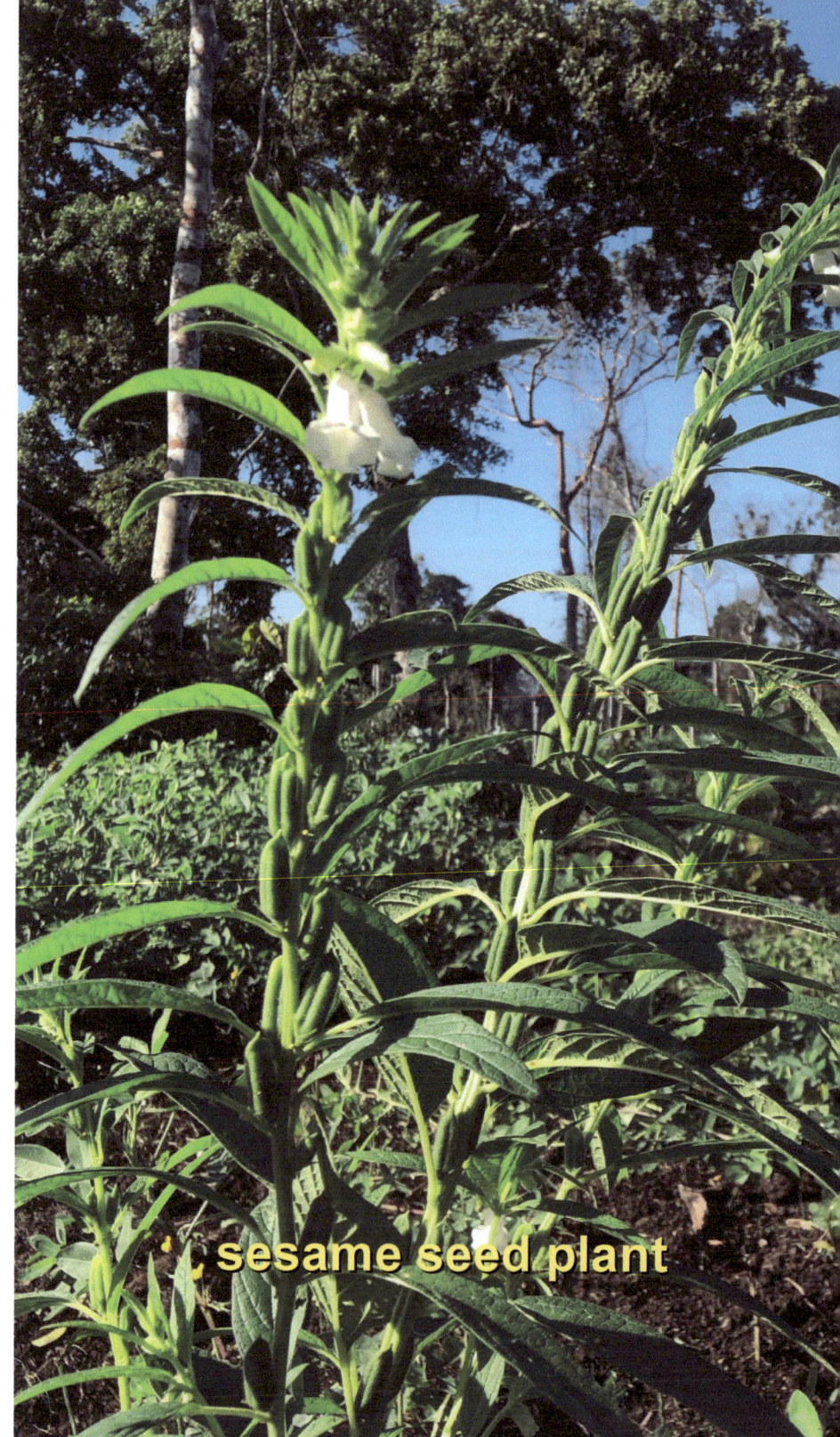

sesame seed plant

Zinc

Zinc is one of the minerals in food that has received the most attention for its ability to support immune function. Zinc is an essential mineral involved in the production of certain immune cells. Zinc develops and activates T-lymphocytes (T-cells) and helps prevent cold viruses from binding and replicating in the mucous membranes of the nose. The National Institutes of Health (NIH) caution that even mildly low levels of zinc may impair your immune function. The mineral zinc is also involved in producing serotonin, as well as hundreds of other brain pathways. Zinc is noted as being essential to learning: it is used in the growth of nerve cells, and it also aids in making new connections between nerve cells. In addition, zinc is essential in the formation of memory, and is found abundantly in the area of the brain responsible for processing short-term and long-term memory.

Here are some top food sources of zinc: nuts, pumpkin seeds, sesame seeds, beans, and lentils.

Maintaining adequate but not excessive levels of zinc is important. This is one reason food is such an excellent source of obtaining nutrition versus supplementation; food contains a balanced variety of the micronutrients whereas supplementation with individual nutrients can lead to too much of some and not enough of others.

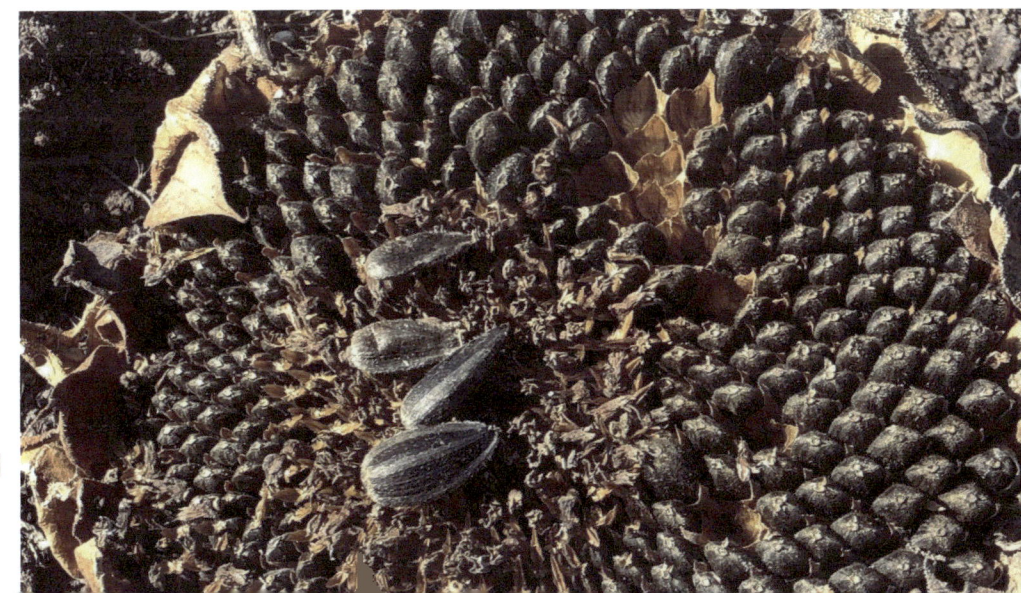

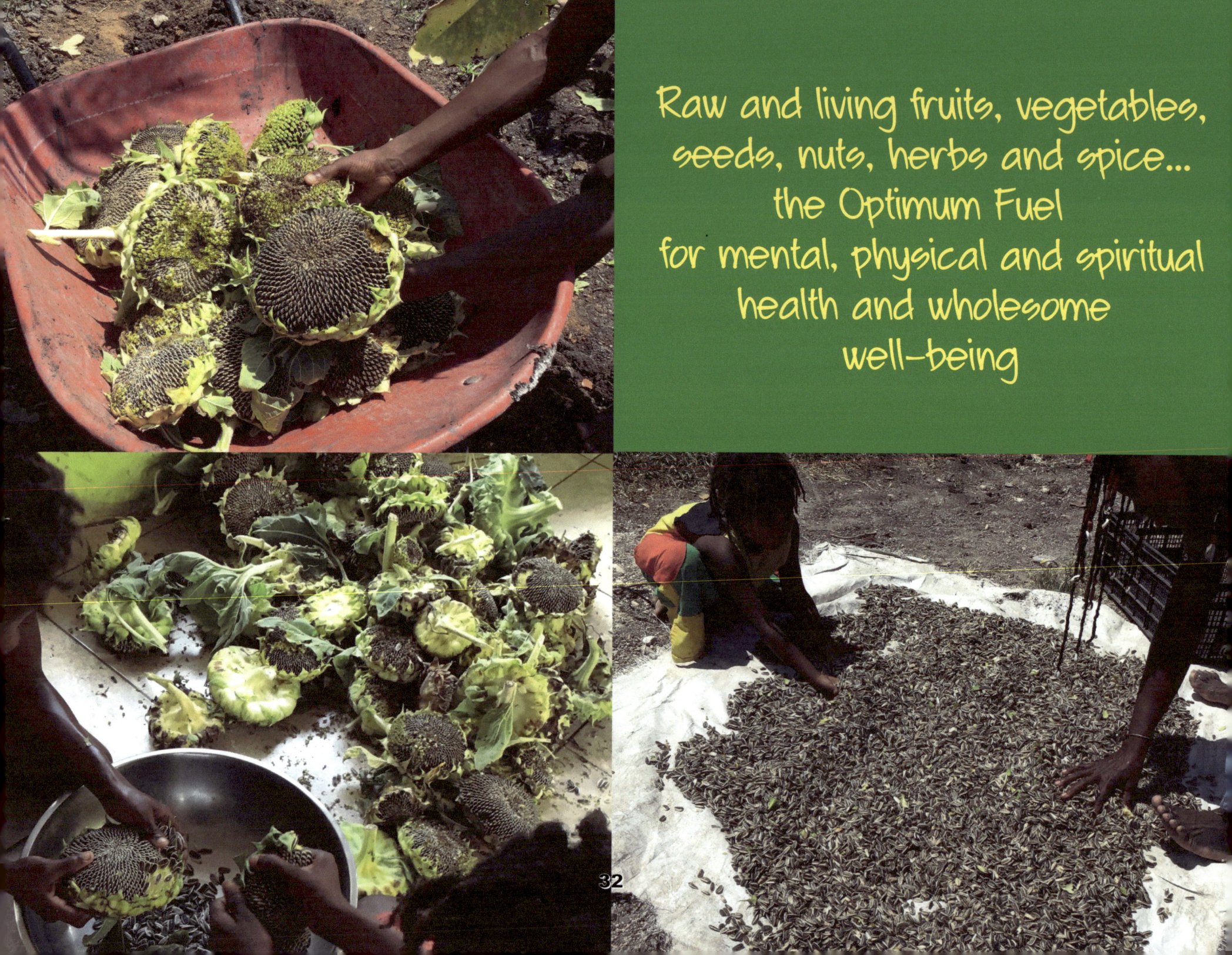

Raw and living fruits, vegetables, seeds, nuts, herbs and spice... the Optimum Fuel for mental, physical and spiritual health and wholesome well-being

CHAPTER 3: DID YOU EAT YOUR GREENS?

A point to remember is that fruits cleanse and vegetables repair. As a general group, green leafy vegetables are potent body healers and help to rebuild the cell structure of the body. We say that raw and living fruits, vegetables, seeds and nuts are the way to go. While the USDA recommendation gives a range of 5 to 6 cups of fruits and vegetables each day as a standard consumption pattern, we say take it to the max. Fuel your body with optimum nutrition for optimum mental, physical and spiritual health and well-being.

Green leafy vegetables like kale, collards, spinach, chard, turnip greens, bok choy, and broccoli rabe are an excellent source of vitamins, minerals and antioxidants. In fact, green leafy vegetables are one of the best sources of B vitamins. You may have noticed that there is a lot of attention on kale as one of the most nutritious greens.

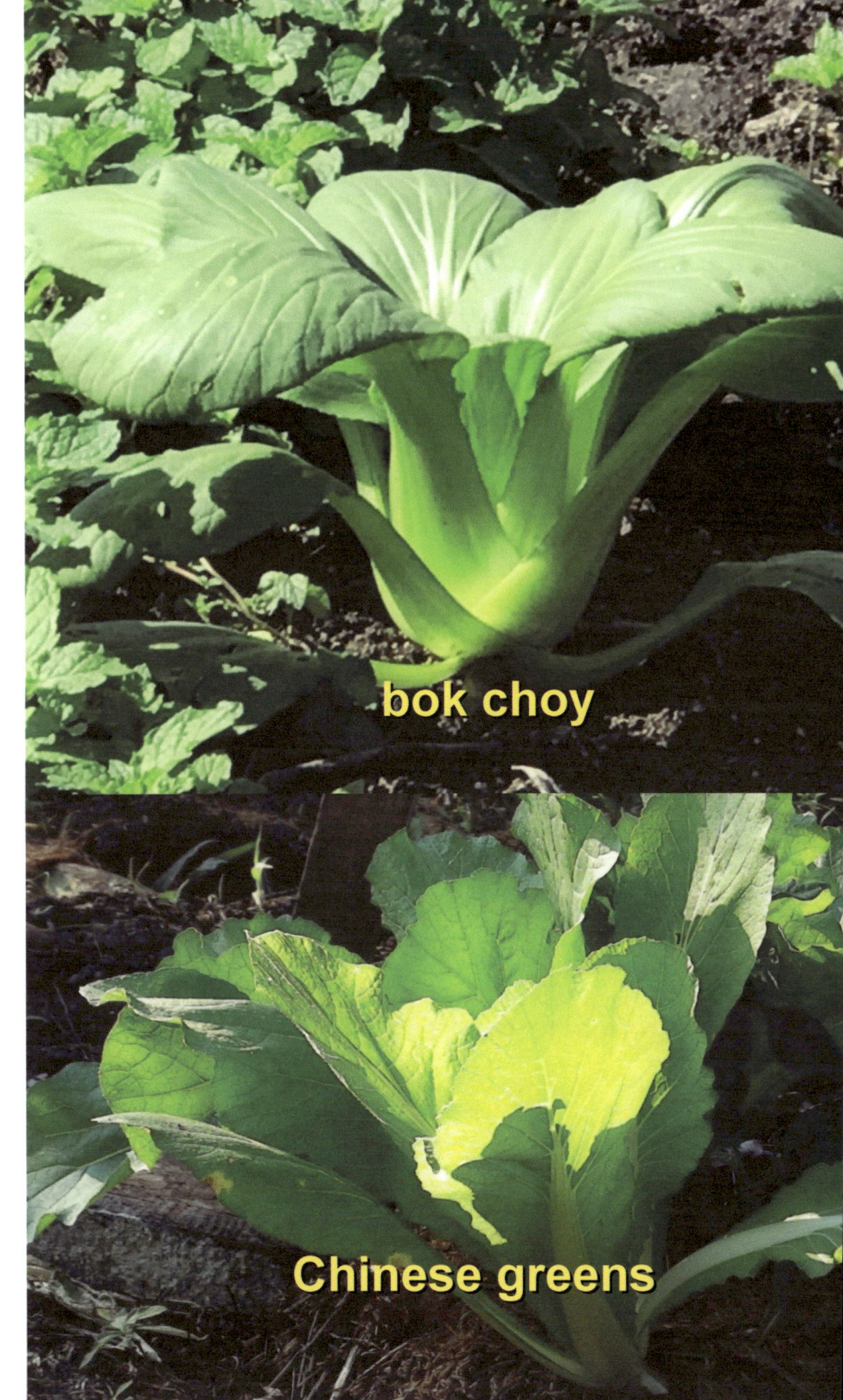
bok choy

Chinese greens

Kale

Kale has been shown to contain high levels of vitamins A (from beta carotene), K, B_6 and C, calcium, potassium, copper and manganese. The truth is, kale is actually one of the world's best sources of vitamin C. A cup of raw kale contains even more vitamin C than a whole orange.

Kale comes in many varieties.

▶Curly kale is the most commonly known and has bright green leaves with curly edges. Our curly kale — Siberian Dwarf variety — is one of the most popular greens we provide at the local farmers' market..

▶Dinosaur kale or, as we refer to it within the Kwatamani First Genesis Tribe, flat leaf kale, has narrow green leaves that are rough and wrinkled. The leaves are attached to a firm stem.

▶Premiere kale has ruffled leaves with rich green color.

▶Purple kale has a deep red to purple stem.

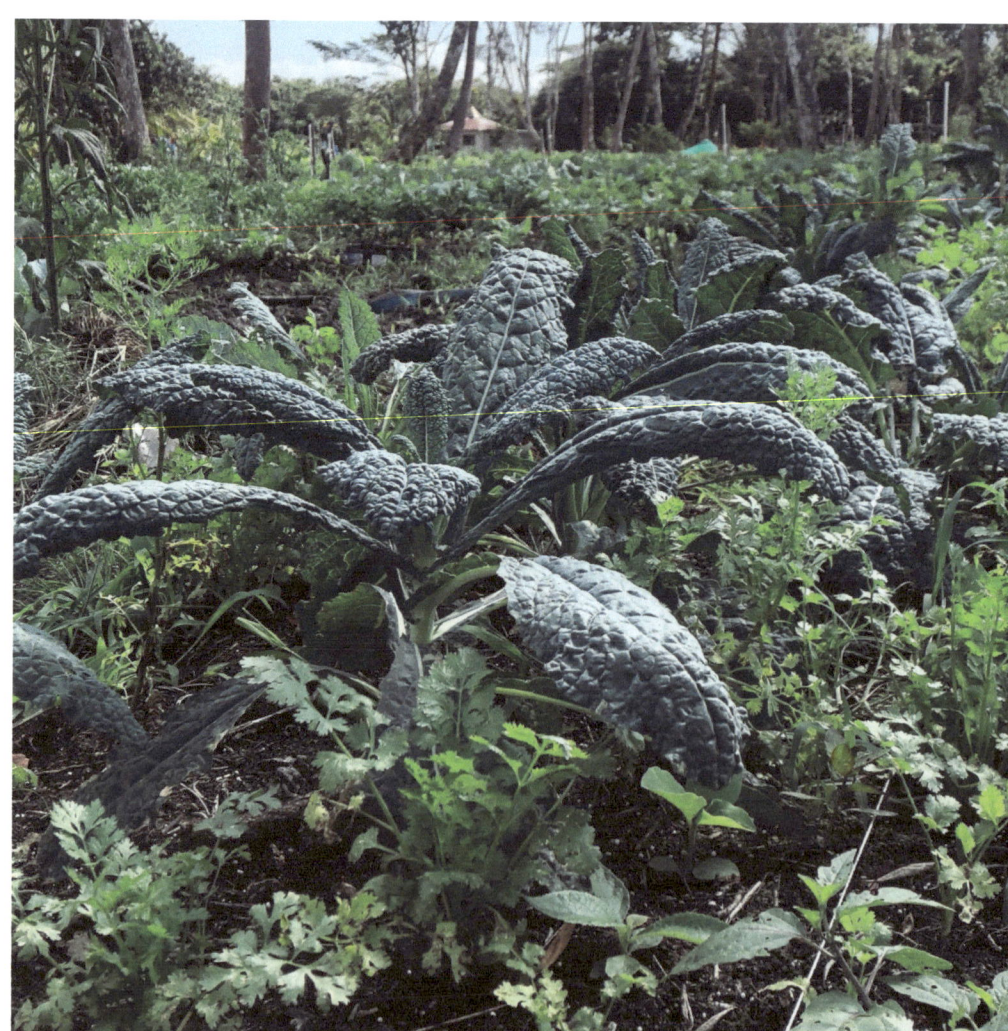

Curly kale has a crunchy, crisp texture and is excellent with a salad dressing on top.

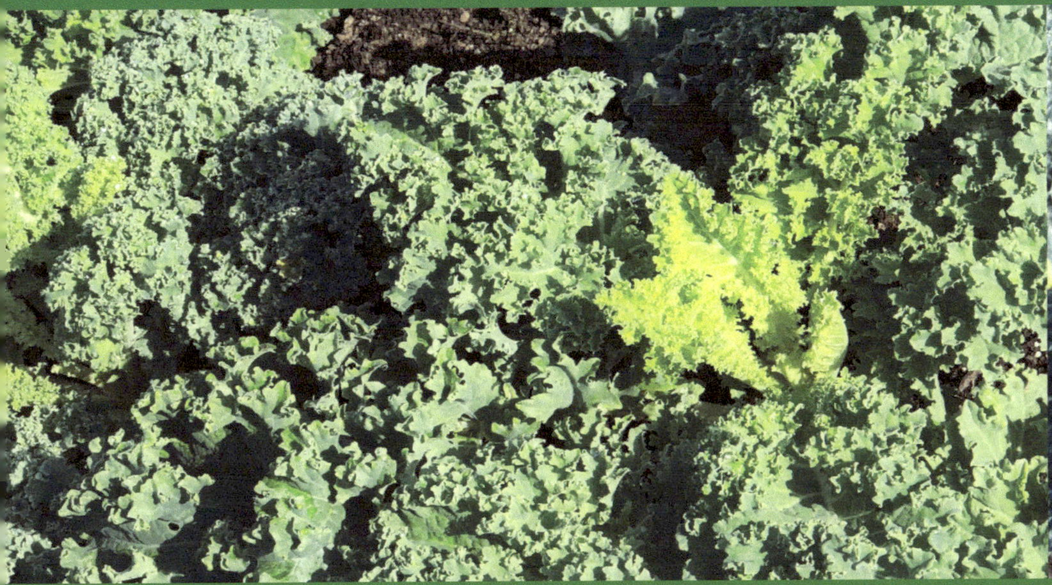

Dinosaur kale is a deep, dark green with robust flavor that mixes well in green juice blends.

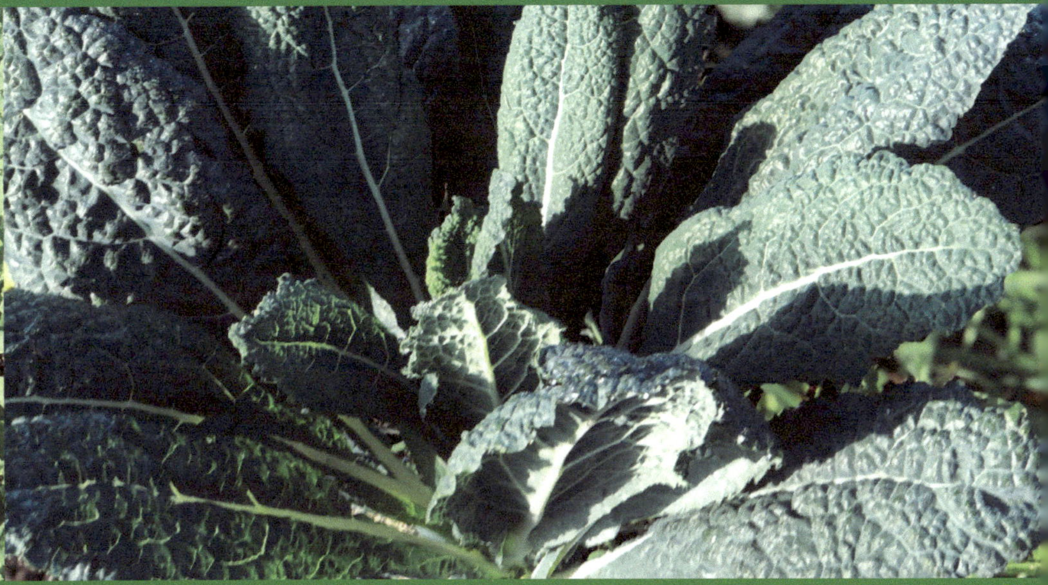

Premiere kale is tender with a mild flavor, making it a favorite in marinated greens dishes.

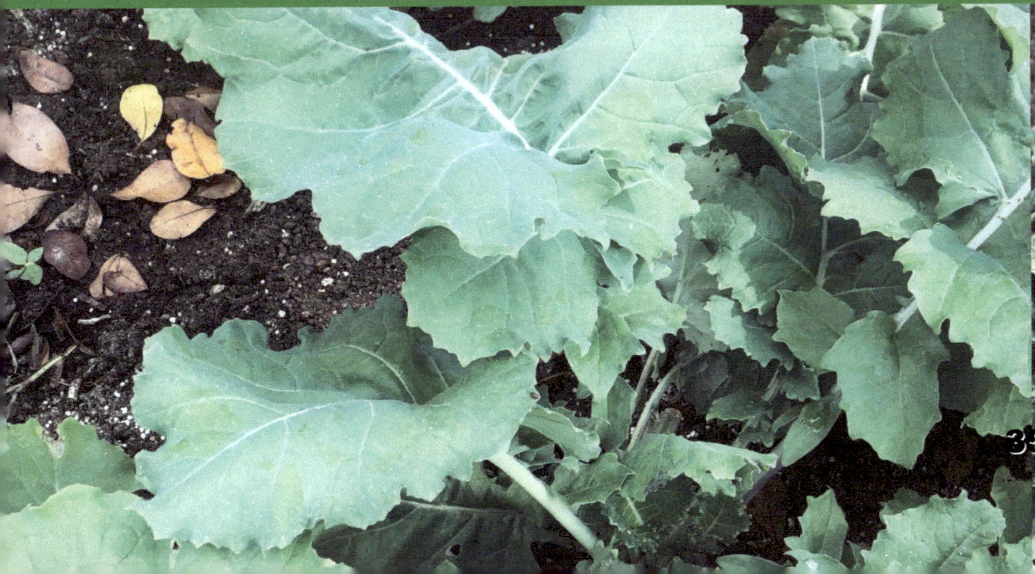

Purple kale has a soft texture and mild flavor that mixes well with other greens.

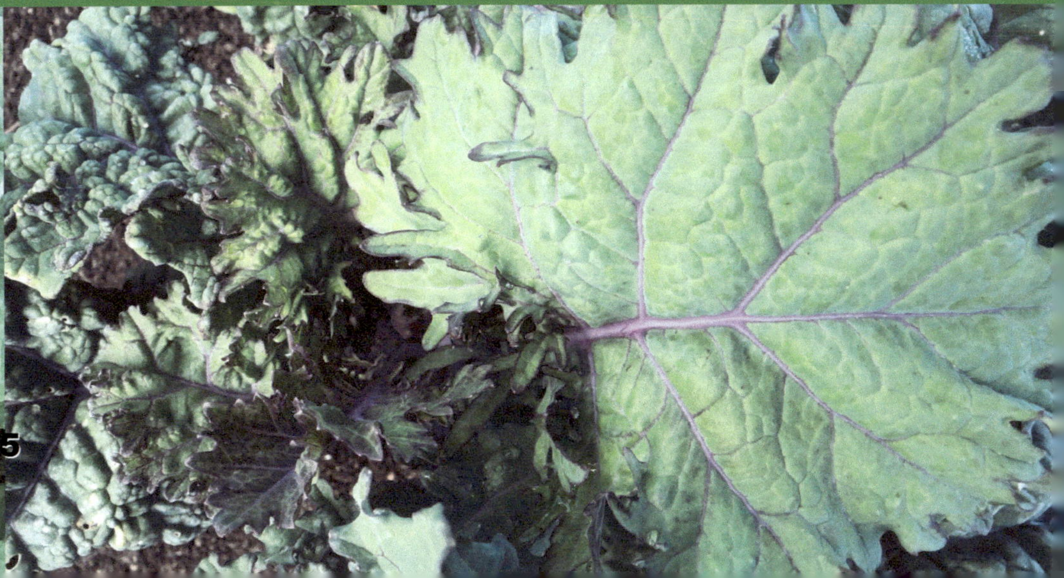

Vates Blue Curled Kale has a
sturdy leaf texture
with a slighty nutty flavor.

Our year-and-a-half-old granddaughter enjoys
sharing a plate of kale salad with grandpa
every chance she gets.
Remember children learn by example.

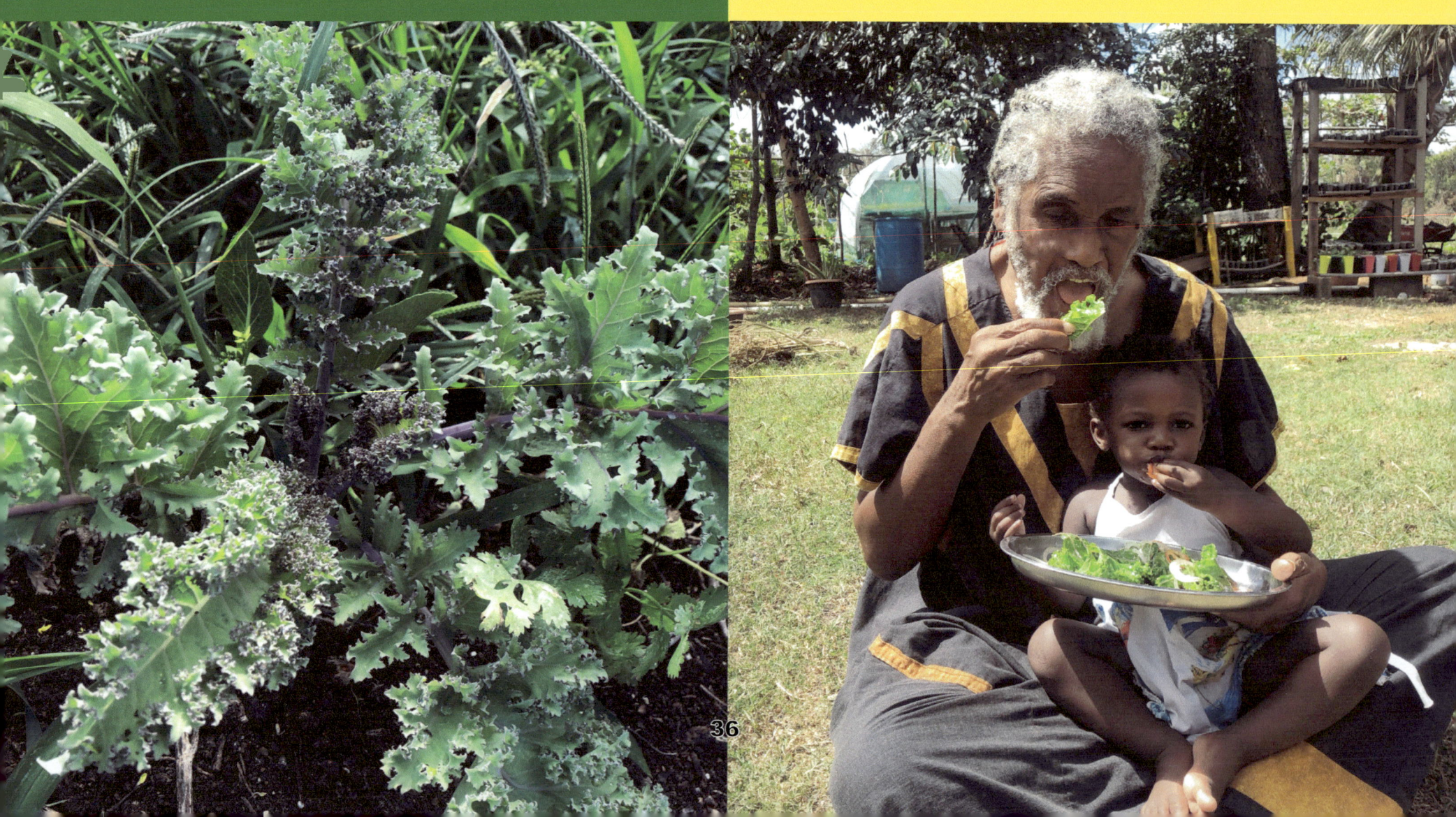

CHAPTER 3: DID YOU EAT YOUR GREENS?

It is true that vegetables contain nutrients that can provide health benefits and the cruciferous vegetables as a group are highly potent. Cruciferous vegetables, plants of the cabbage family, are powerful immune-boosting vegetables. These vegetables have a chemical composition that includes sulfur. The sulfur they contain is responsible for their strong distinct flavor. When these vegetables are broken down by biting, blending, or chopping, a chemical reaction occurs that converts the sulfur-containing compounds into a powerful substance that has been shown to help prevent and neutralize cancer and has proven immune-boosting capabilities.

Cruciferous vegetables contain antiviral and antibacterial agents that help maintain a disease-free state of being. Let your daily plate of delicious fresh, raw/uncooked greens provide that immunity enhancement that helps to naturally ward off infectious disease.

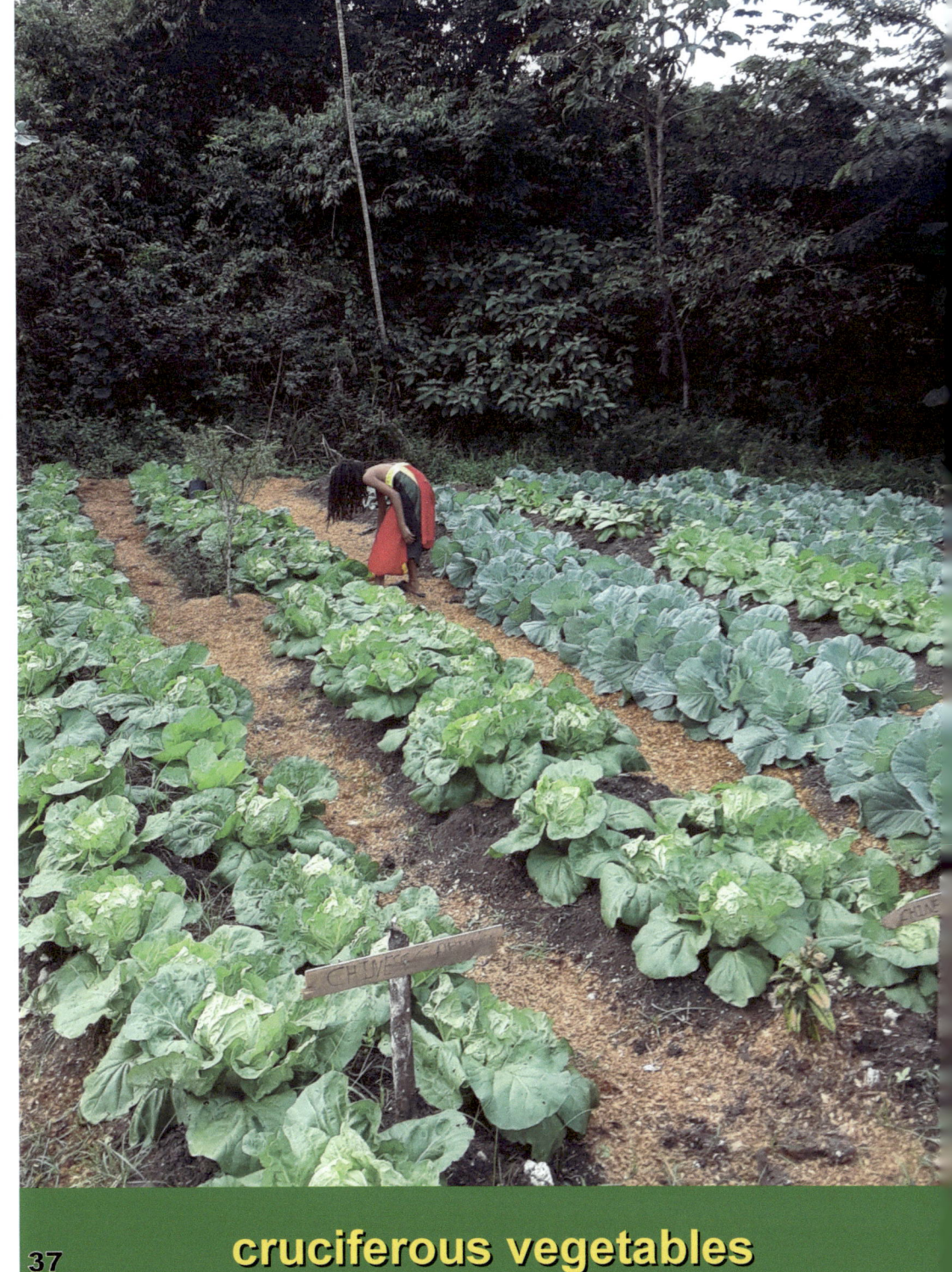

cruciferous vegetables

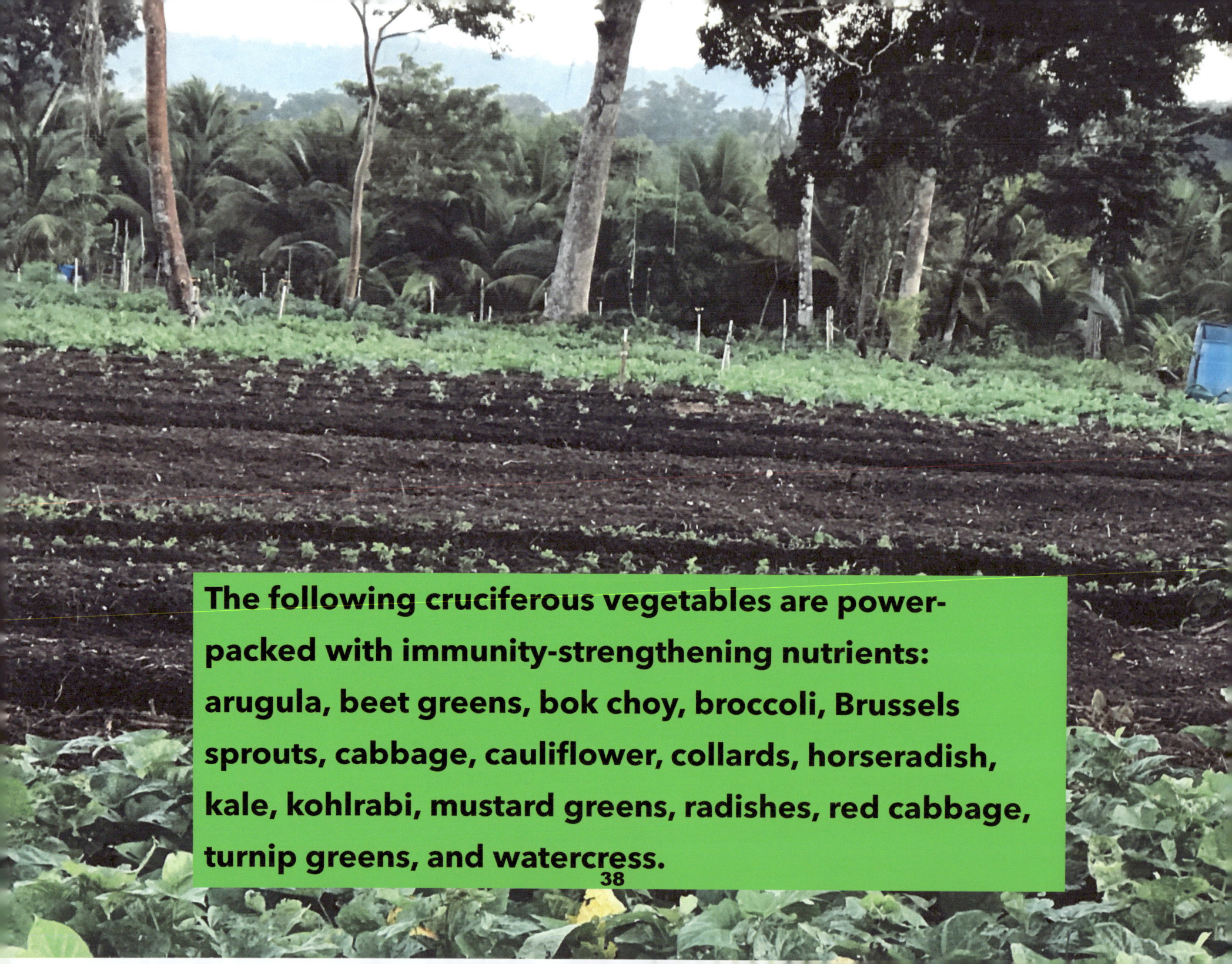

The following cruciferous vegetables are power-packed with immunity-strengthening nutrients: arugula, beet greens, bok choy, broccoli, Brussels sprouts, cabbage, cauliflower, collards, horseradish, kale, kohlrabi, mustard greens, radishes, red cabbage, turnip greens, and watercress.

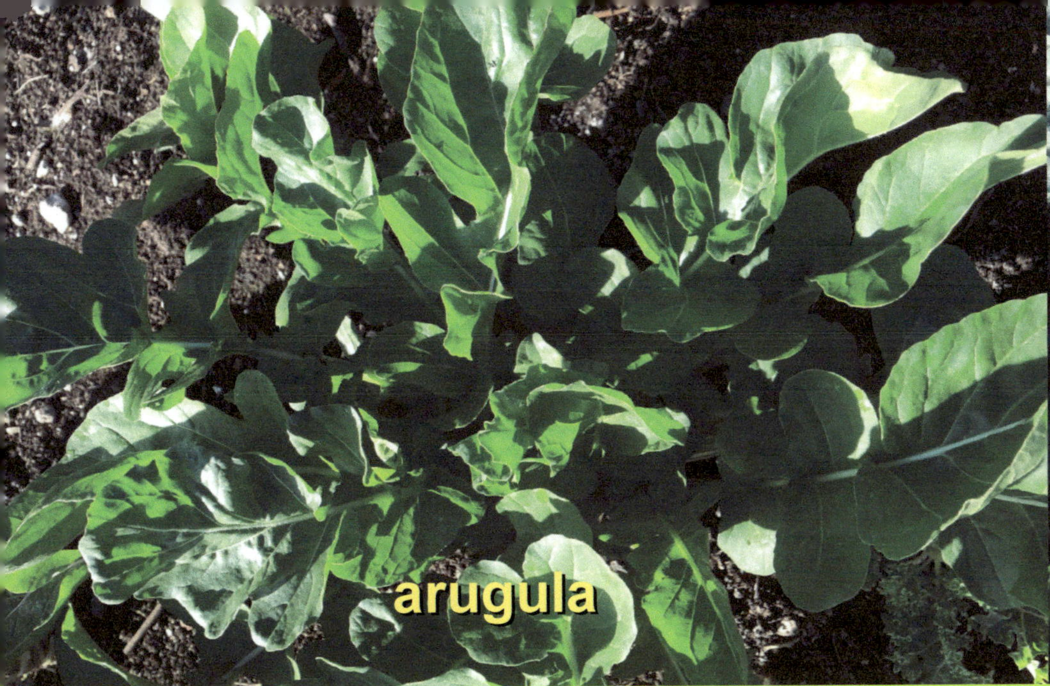

arugula

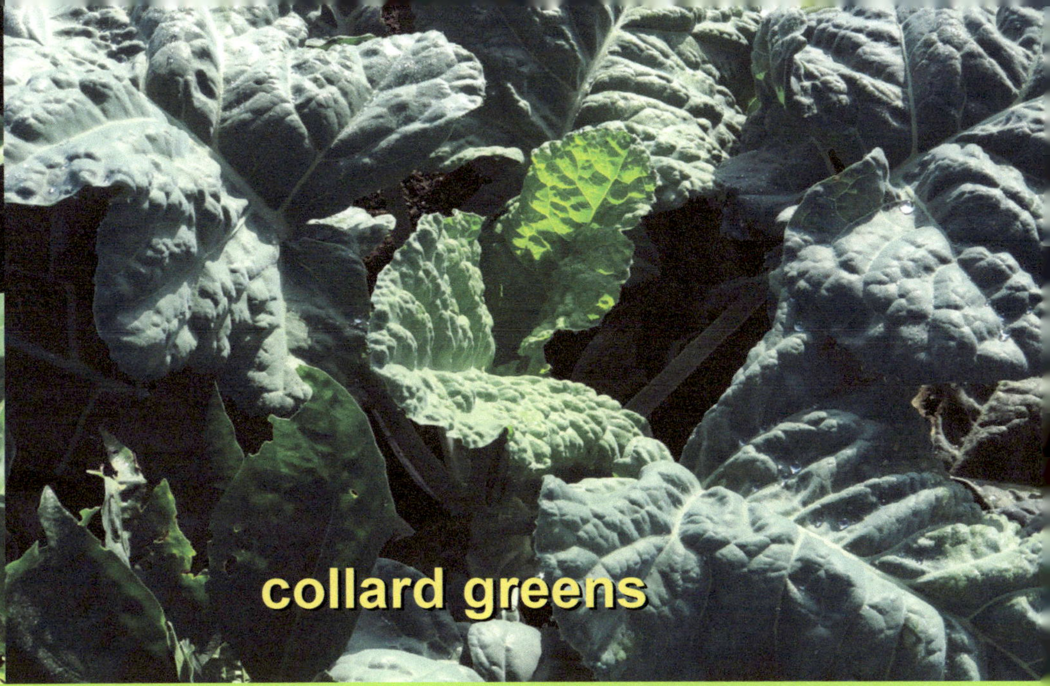

collard greens

Of the physical barriers that protect your internal organs from any pathogens in the outside world, your gastrointestinal tract is of primary importance. The gastrointestinal tract is like an internal skin, but it has about 150 times more surface than does your outside skin. It also contains the largest number of immune cells of your whole body, constituting approximately 60% of your entire immune system.

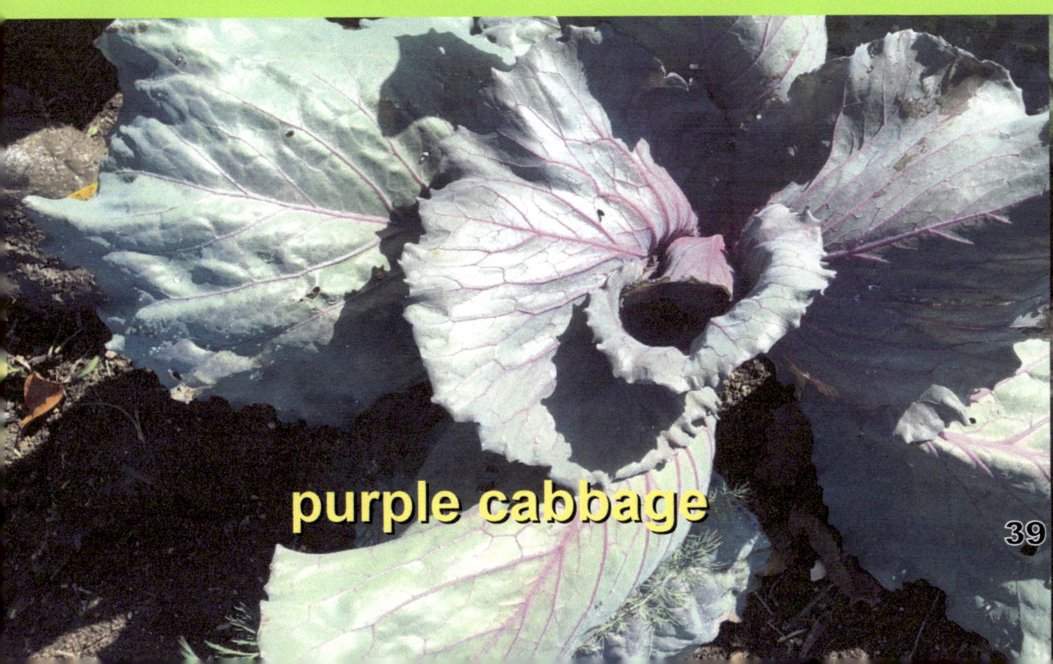

purple cabbage

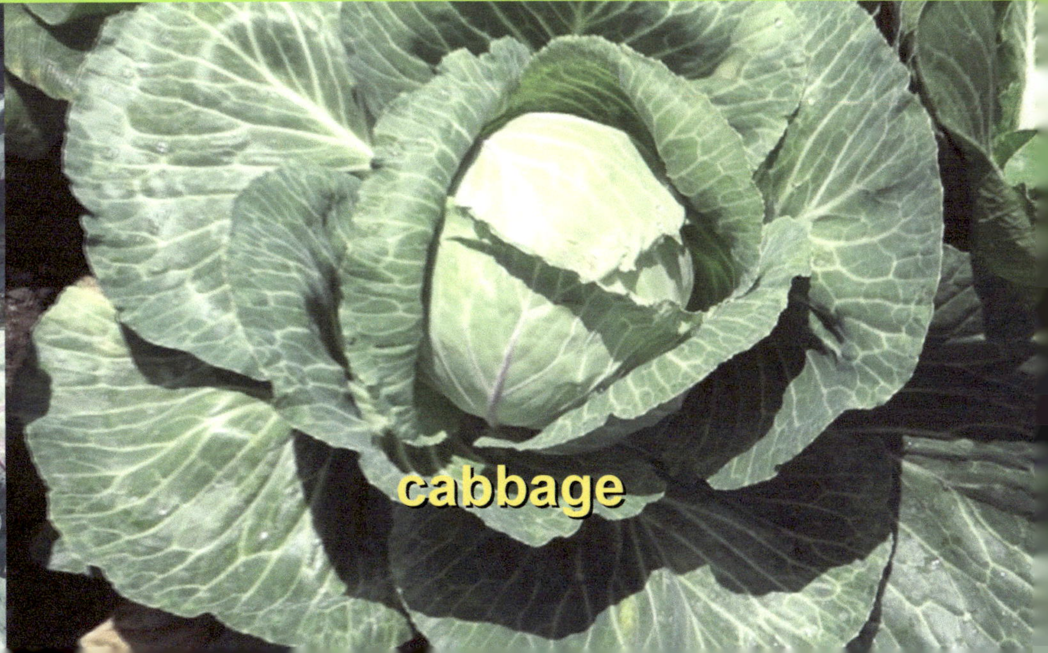

cabbage

Lettuce

Each kind of lettuce provides a high level of antioxidants, water, fiber and essential nutrients. Lettuce contains minerals such as potassium, calcium, and magnesium. Leaf lettuce grows from a single stalk while "head" lettuce grows in a ball-like cluster.

A recent study published in Neurology found that those who ate the most leafy greens each day had slower rates of mental decline compared to those who ate the least. Remember that the brain needs to be nourished in order to safeguard mental immunity.

Beta-carotene, the plant pigment that is normally associated with carrots and other yellow orange vegetables, is also hiding in leafy greens. Think of autumn leaves changing colors. As they lose chlorophyll (the pigment that makes them green), you can see the red, orange, and yellow pigments those leaves contain underneath. These vibrant colors are also responsible for the potent health benefits of leafy greens. Instead of plain salad with the common iceberg lettuce, we are showing just a few of the lettuce varieties that are growing in our organic/veganic garden. The blends of delicate flavors and crisp to tender textures will certainly make a delicious, quick and simple dish topped with a fresh herbal dressing.

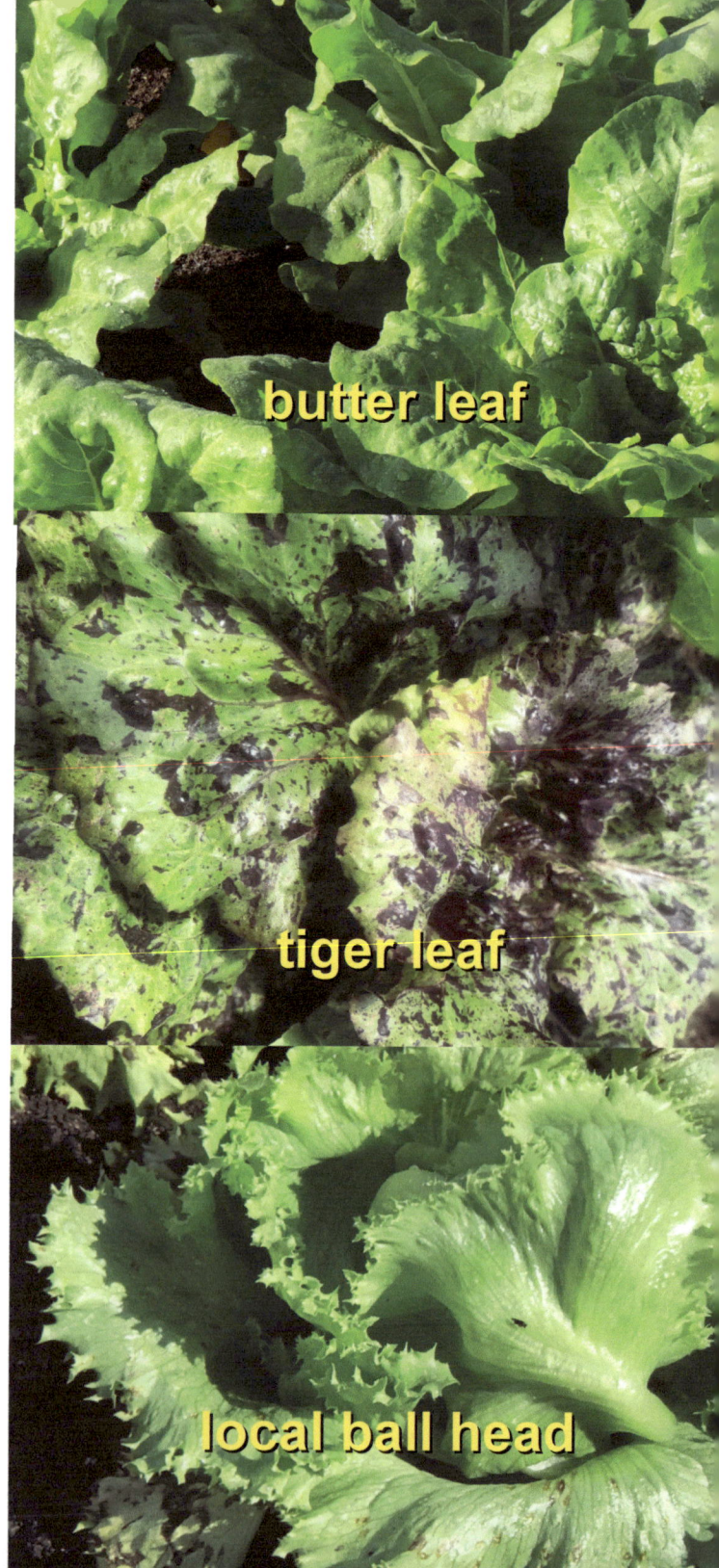

butter leaf

tiger leaf

local ball head

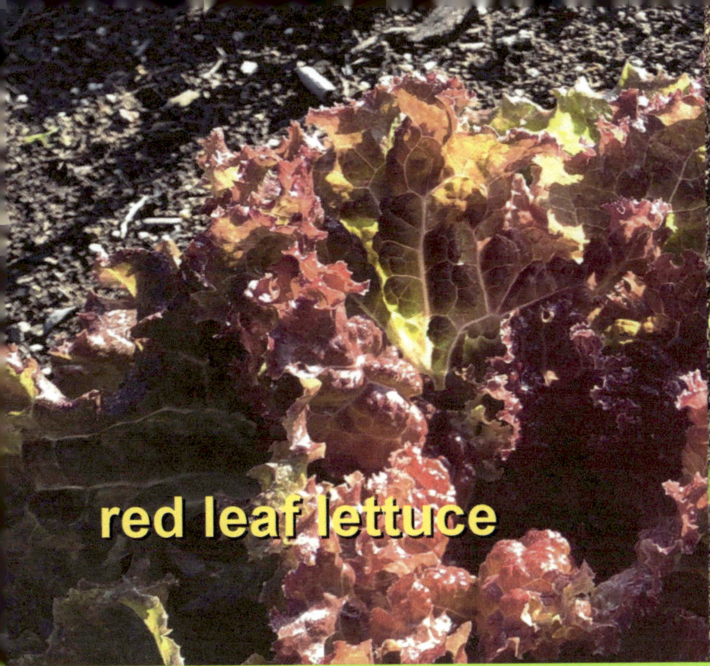

red leaf lettuce

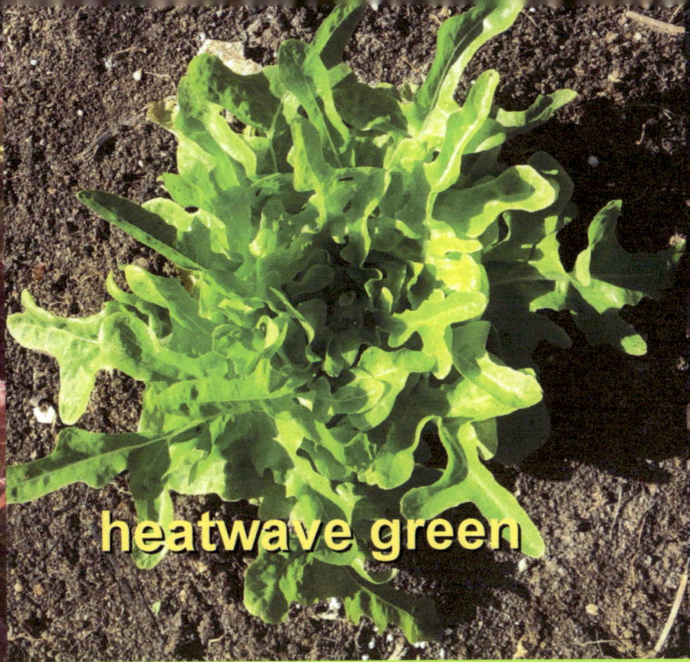

heatwave green

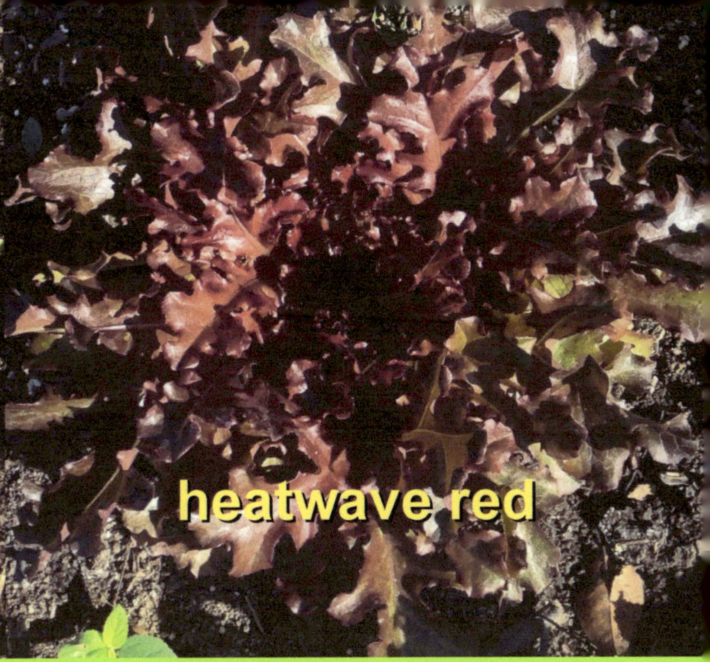

heatwave red

Assorted varieties of lettuce, growing in our veganic/organic garden. We note that many nutritionists identify red leaf lettuces as loaded with more phytonutrients than green leaf lettuce. Phytonutrients are important since they give lettuce its red color and are loaded with antioxidant properties needed to build a strong immune system. For this reason red leaf lettuce is considered the healthiest type of lettuce.

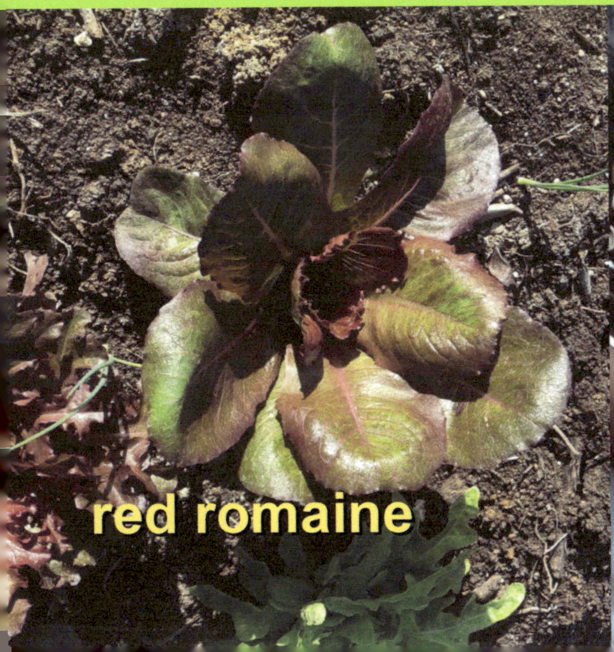

red romaine

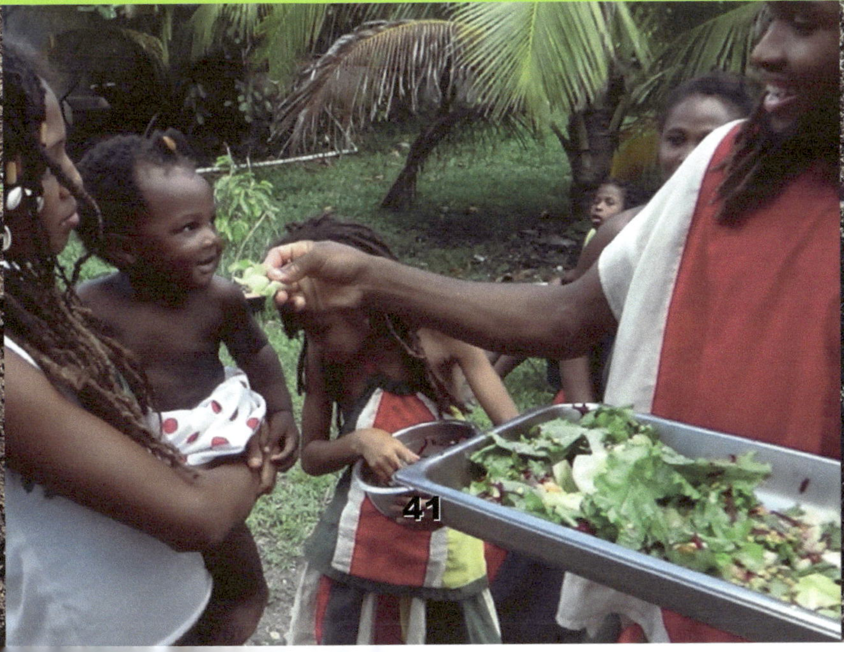

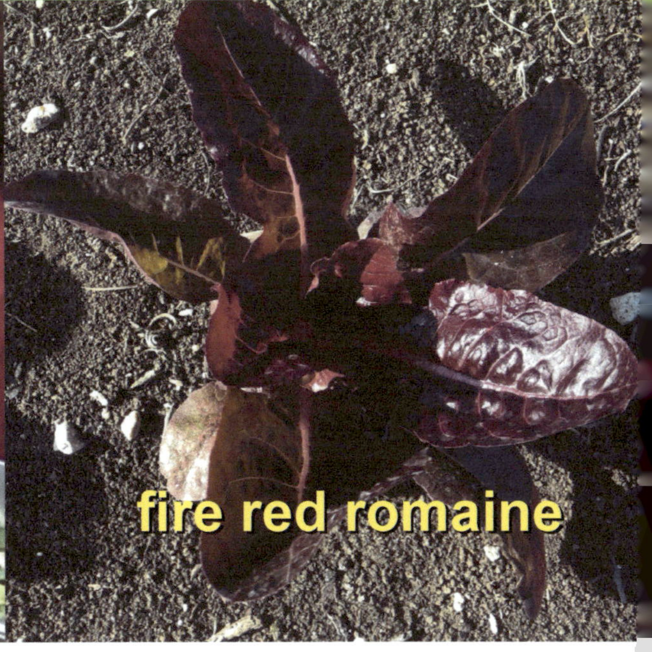

fire red romaine

Nutrition

continues to be a major
determining factor in the survival
of the human species.
High Priest Kwatamani, KRIST Text, p. 140

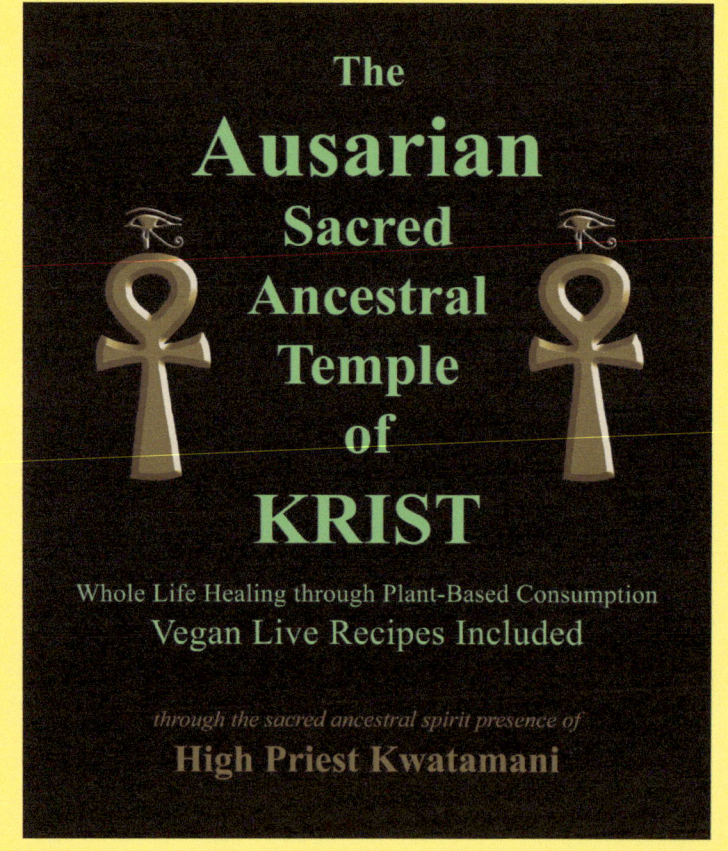

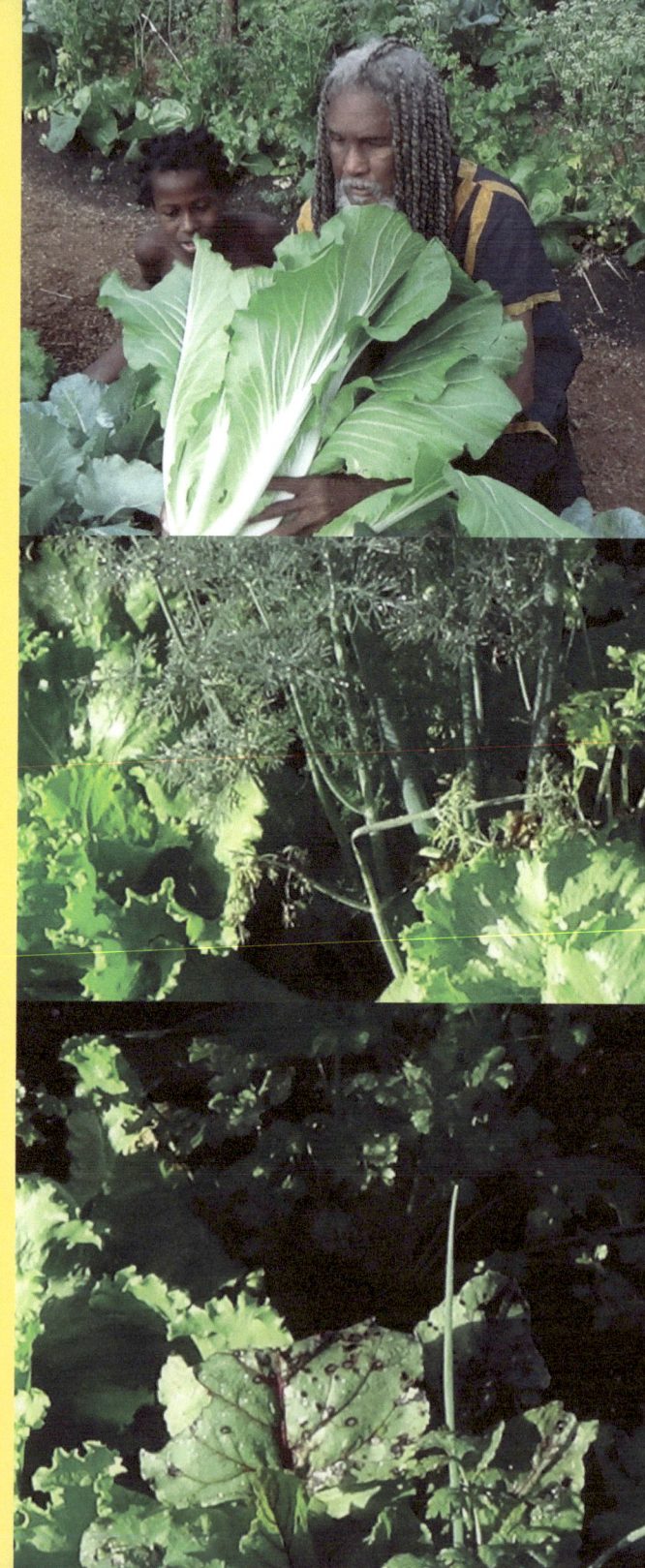

CHAPTER 4: THE BEST DEFENSE

FRESH FROM THE GARDEN

The I in I have been inspired for over 55 years to honor and glorify the magnificence of raw and living fruits, vegetables, seeds, and nuts by creating some of the most enjoyable, pleasurable, and stimulating live vegan meals imaginable. And the first ingredient is divine humility to the Supreme Essence of earth, wind, rain, and sun. From there, inspiration flows from one's own spirit-conscious desire to celebrate the colors, smells, textures, flavors, and taste sensations from the garden while tuning in to the variety of nutrient and energy factors provided.

We are sure that you will find in transitioning to a live foods diet that your taste buds will begin to alter. When consuming a dead and devitalized diet, the taste buds become dulled by excessive salt, artificial flavors, artificial colors, additives, preservatives, processed starches and flours, cooked foods and excess and artificial sugars in

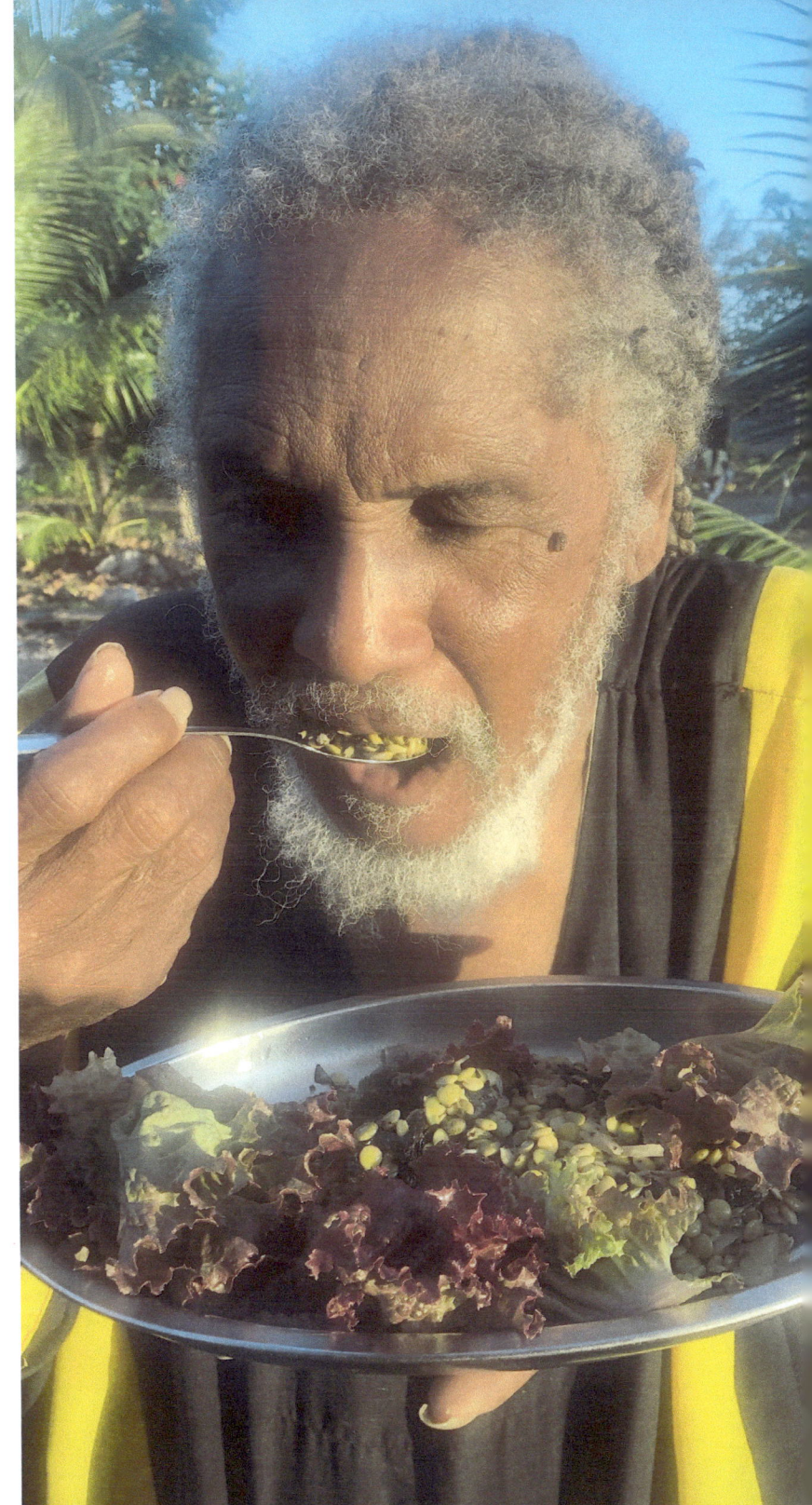

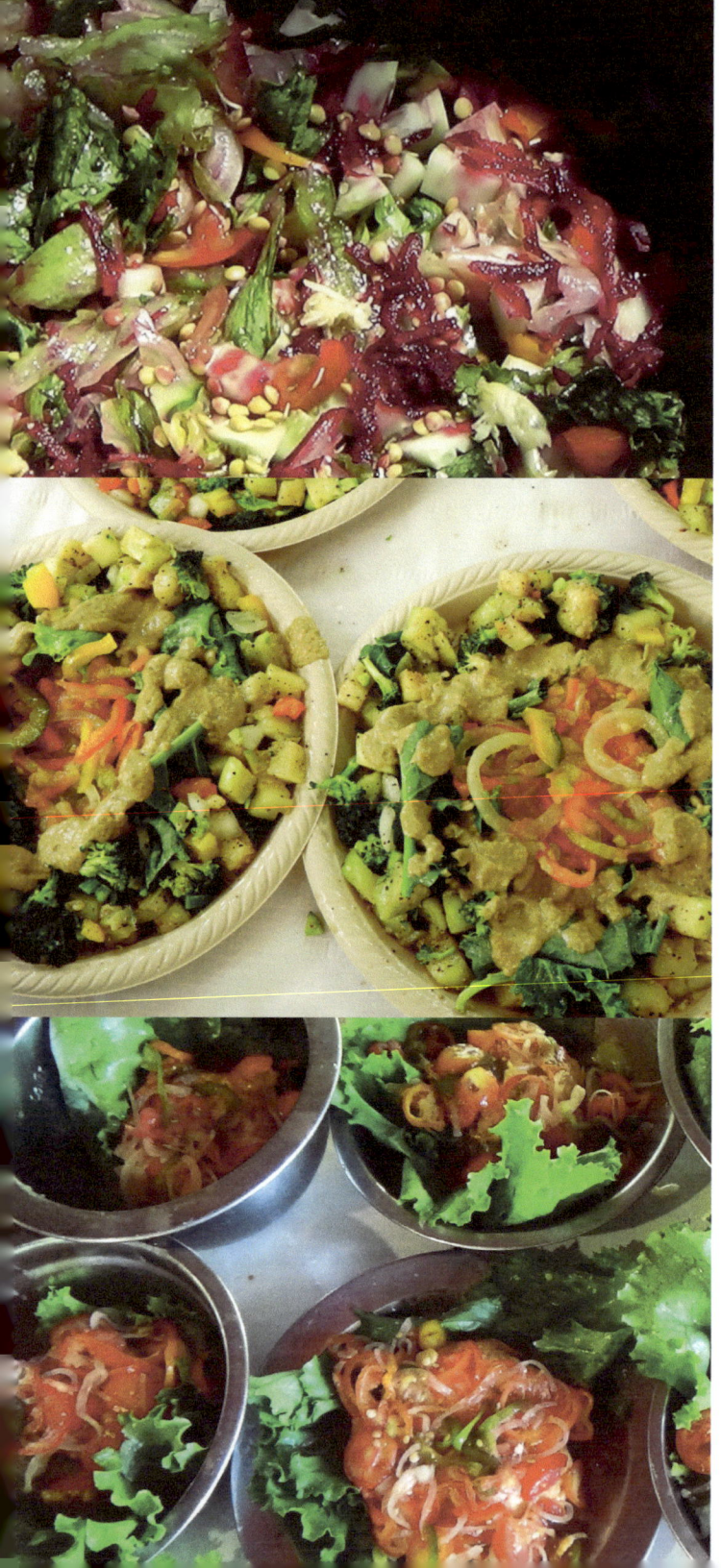

the diet. As you become accustomed to consuming only live and whole foods, your natural taste buds will become enhanced, and you will develop a deep love and appreciation for fresh, live and whole fruits, vegetables, seeds, nuts and grains in their raw, living and natural state.

Our approach to food preparation is that all foods and meals are combined and prepared for maximum digestibility and nutritive value. Rather than giving you a list of recipes with measurements and minutia, our purpose is to equip you with the knowledge and basic understanding of the foods and how they are best combined for maximum health and flavor. This information will include suggested food combinations and slicing and marinating techniques. You can then get creative, applying these principles and techniques in exciting and innumerable ways.

These recipes will set the pace for an entirely new way of "LIFE" live food preparation. It is the intent of the Kwatamani First Genesis Tribe to teach you how to innercourse with live foods instead of giving you a large quantity of bland recipes that we no longer use. These are traditional Kwatamani recipes.

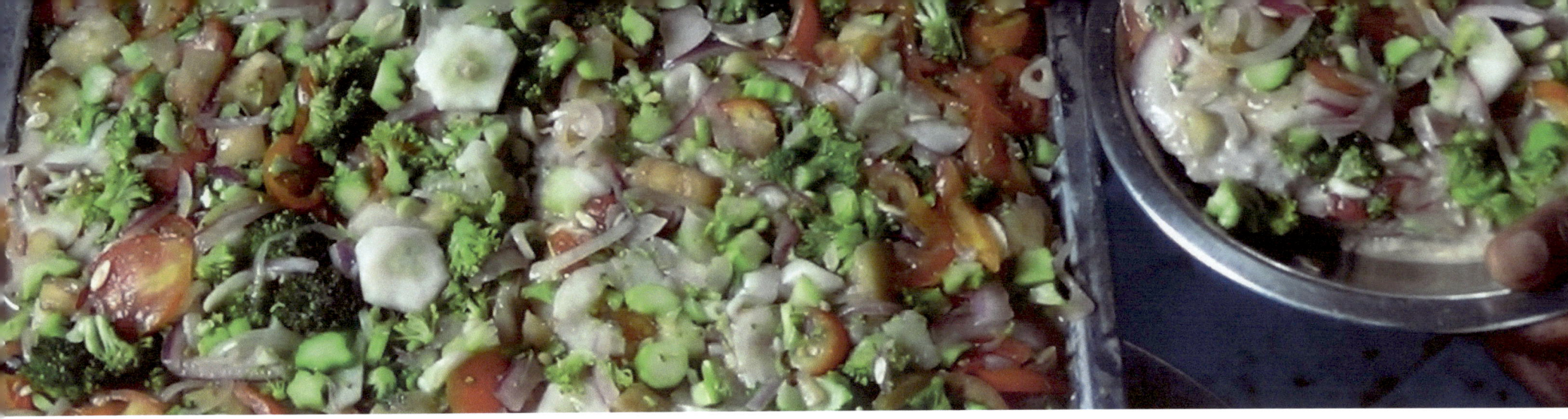

Some basic equipment:

- Sharp, stainless steel knives

- Garlic press or grater. Used to press or grate fresh garlic cloves. Avoid the cheap plastic varieties. Look for the sturdy stainless steel ones. Pressing or grating the garlic improves its taste and digestibility.

- Food Processor . We recommend the Cuisinart. The food processor can be used for grinding nuts and making puddings, cakes, pie crusts and purees. Raw and Living Foods, p. 131.

All vegetables in the recipes should be washed clean and ready to eat.

We tend to use fresh coconut oil, because we have lots of coconut trees. However, flaxseed oil is very beneficial to use, as well as first cold-pressed extra virgin olive oil if the other two are not available. As far as the measurements for the ingredients in each recipe, we tend to use quantities in relationship to one's body proportions. For example, one should use one's hand as the measuring cup to prepare a single serving size for any dish. Thus, a fruit or vegetable the size of one's fist would be considered as the average size. Using a handful of nuts or the amount of greens that one can hold in one hand would be the proportion for a single serving.

For juices and other liquids, the amount of liquid that can be held in one's cupped palm would be the average amount. One could easily multiply the number of handfuls used based on the number of people one would be serving and the size of one's appetite.

The featured recipes in this text are representative of the many fruits, vegetables, seeds, and nuts that one can use in many different combinations to create many different nutritious and delicious dishes. Raw and living fruits, vegetables, seeds, and nuts provide a wide variety of essential nutrient elements which enhance one's physical strength, endurance, agility, coordination, and immune defense system.

The bright, vibrant colors, curved shapes, and succulent juicy or creamy soft textures of many fruits are naturally pleasing. Yes, the fruits are a sweet favorite, but right now we are going to focus on the vegetation elements of the Tree of Life. Our approach is to consume a variety in abundance; which is reflected throughout the garden, the rain forest, and the natural habitat designed for Man, He and She, and for spiritual alignment. We consume based on the growing season, and this annual rotation of harvest does provide a wonderful selection of raw and living fruits, vegetables, seeds, and nuts.

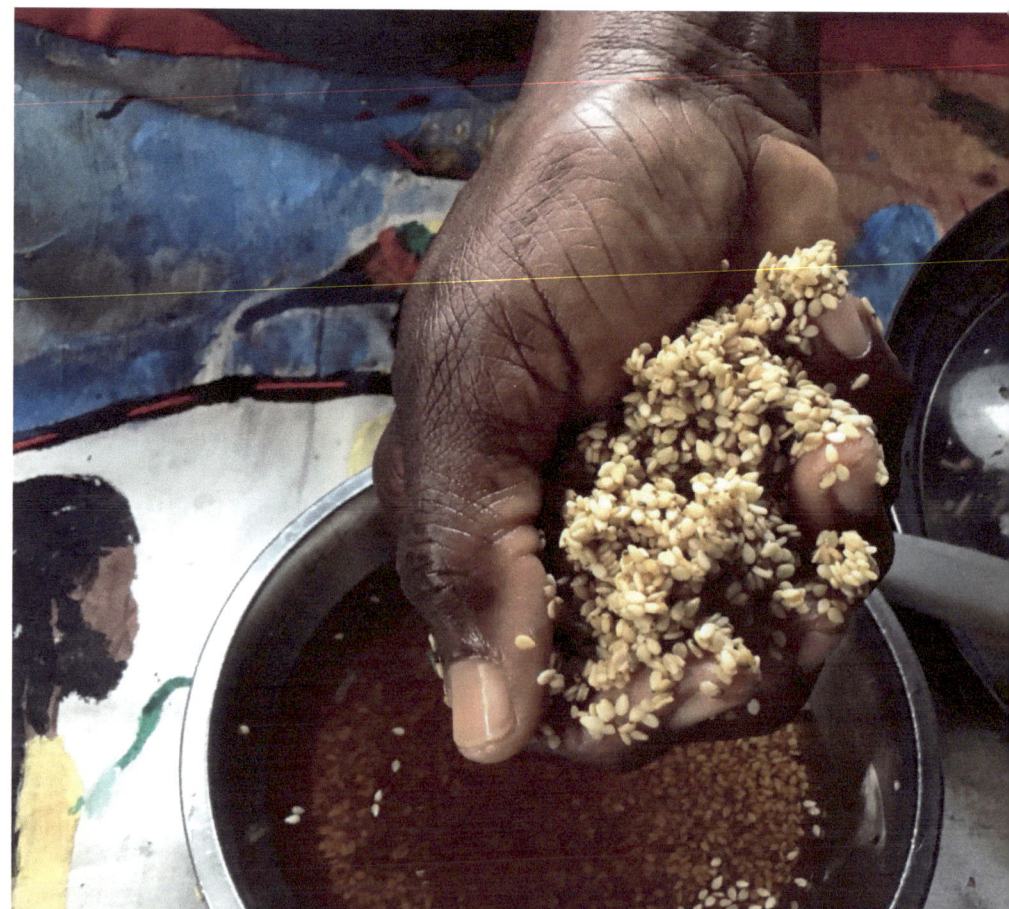

CHAPTER 5: BACK TO BASICS

We include the nutritional values and healing factors of these ingredients so that one may become more aware that every act of consumption can be a life-affirming expression of tender-loving care for one's own being. Plant nutrition is indeed our medicine.

Our daily meals contain various combinations of these basic ingredients. The popular recipes featured in this text are rich with the beneficial nutrients provided by raw and living fruits, vegetables, seeds and nuts as the root, base and foundation of health-conscious consumption.

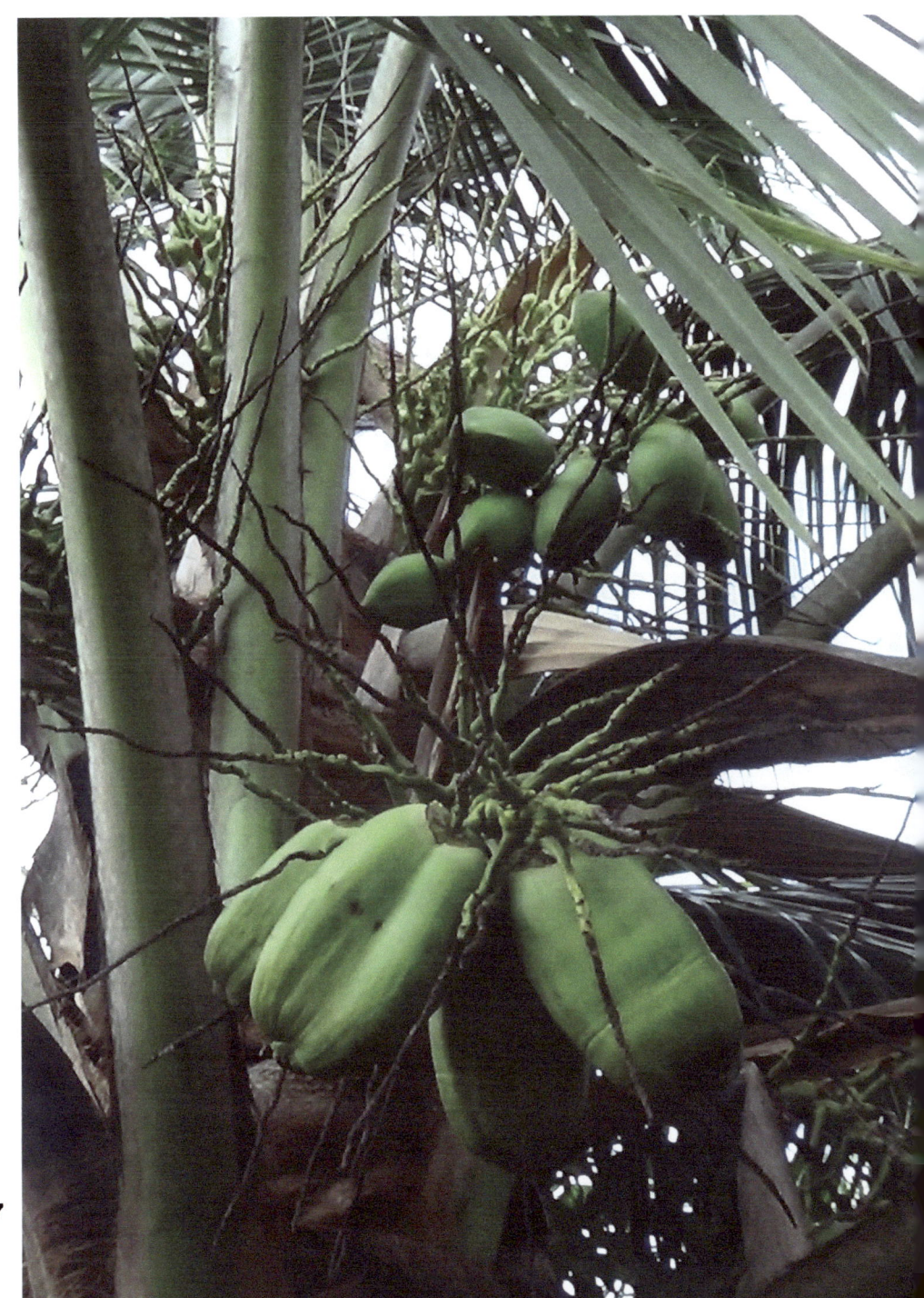

Nourishing whole health

SUPER FOODS

Some of the basic ingredients we use:

coconuts

tomatoes

celery

bell peppers

onion

garlic

limes

Coconuts

Coconuts are fruits and seeds in and of themselves. They are extra special whole foods. Coconuts contain healthy quantities of vitamins B_1 (thiamine), B_2, B_3 and C, calcium, iodine, magnesium, potassium, phosphorus and iron. Coconut is an excellent intestinal cleanser and body builder. It is good for digestive ailments, including stomach ulcers and constipation.

Coconuts alone are capable of wholly nourishing the body. I can recall a time during the war era in West Africa when my family and I lived totally on coconuts, and I can recall other times when we lived solely on sweet and sour sops. These are two fruits that provide all the water or juice content that you need.

Coconuts, as do palm nuts, have the capacity to maintain, build and supply all of the food nourishment needed by the body. Not only is coconut a very wholesome food, it has many other practical uses for body care, maintenance and even for body protection inside and out.

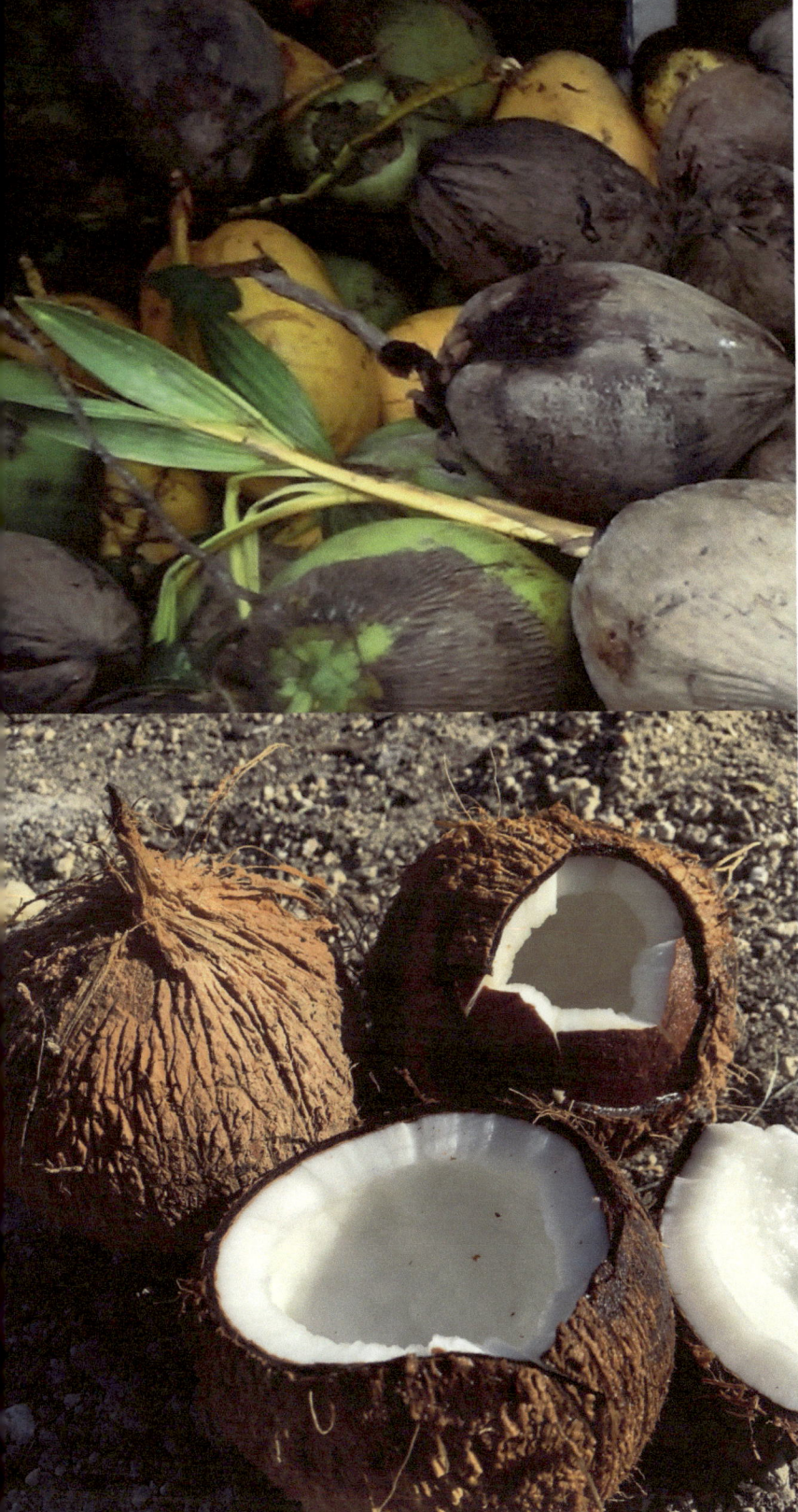

CHAPTER 5: BACK TO THE BASICS

For example, we use the oil to heal cuts, scratches and burns and as a hair and skin oil. Coconut oil can be made right at home by juicing the hard coconut into a milk and letting it sit. Make sure that you drink as much of the milk as possible, because it is an excellent food. In some cases, we have used the coconut milk to feed a child whose mother was unable to breast feed. In fact, coconut milk became primary nourishment for our eldest daughter when we lost her mother just months after her birth during the late '80's Liberian rebel crisis. She is now 32 years-old, birthed as a vegan raw and living foodist, a fully vibrant mated mother of two beautiful offspring. And she says coconuts remain as her favorite whole food.

Remember, when the coconut milk sits for a while, the cream rises to the top, and the oil sits above the cream. We have found coconut oil, coconut cream and coconut milk to be excellent in inspiring hair growth. It best serves you when you take it both internally and externally…As I've said, coconuts are the superfood —one of the few items on this planet that you could eat and receive the bulk of whole living nourishment.
Raw and Living Foods, p. 71.

Tomatoes are definitely a wonder food.

Tomatoes

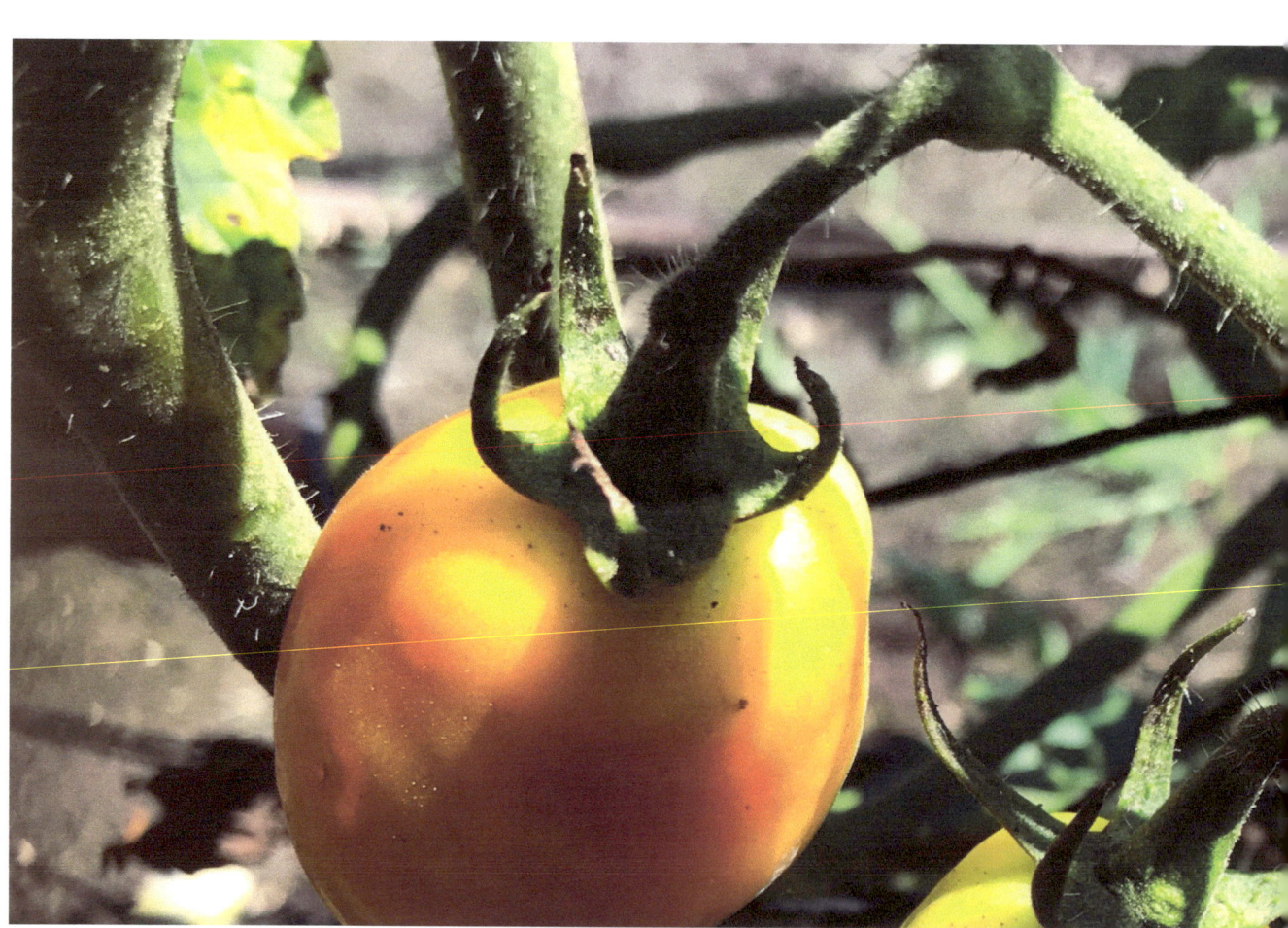

Tomatoes are high in vitamins A and C, biotin, sodium, calcium, potassium, silicon, magnesium and chlorine. Tomatoes also contain inositol, vitamins B_1, B_2, B_3 and K, phosphorus and iron. The tomato is a liver cleanser and stimulates circulation and the heart. It is a natural antiseptic and blood cleanser and purifier, protecting against infection. Tomatoes improve the skin, because they are such good cleansers of toxic waste in the blood. I have used tomatoes or recommended their usage in treating cases of gout, rheumatism, tuberculosis, high blood pressure, high

CHAPTER 5: BACK TO THE BASICS

cholesterol, sinus trouble, liver congestion, gallstones, gas, colds, and obesity. I have received many testimonials over the years about their effectiveness in treating these conditions. I have used the skins, by applying them externally, to treat ringworm, pus-filled sores and acne. The Vitamin K in tomatoes helps to prevent hemorrhages, by aiding in blood clotting. I'm sure that you can see that tomatoes are definitely a wonder food. Tomatoes serve as an internal and external first aid kit and fruit for our household. Someone should have coined the phrase: A tomato a day keeps the doctor away.

Note: As with all foods, tomatoes are very detrimental to the system if eaten cooked, especially when combined with concentrated starches, e.g. combinations like pizza, pasta with tomato sauce, etc. When cooked, tomatoes become acidic, leaching minerals from tissues, teeth and bones. *Raw and Living Foods, p. 84.*

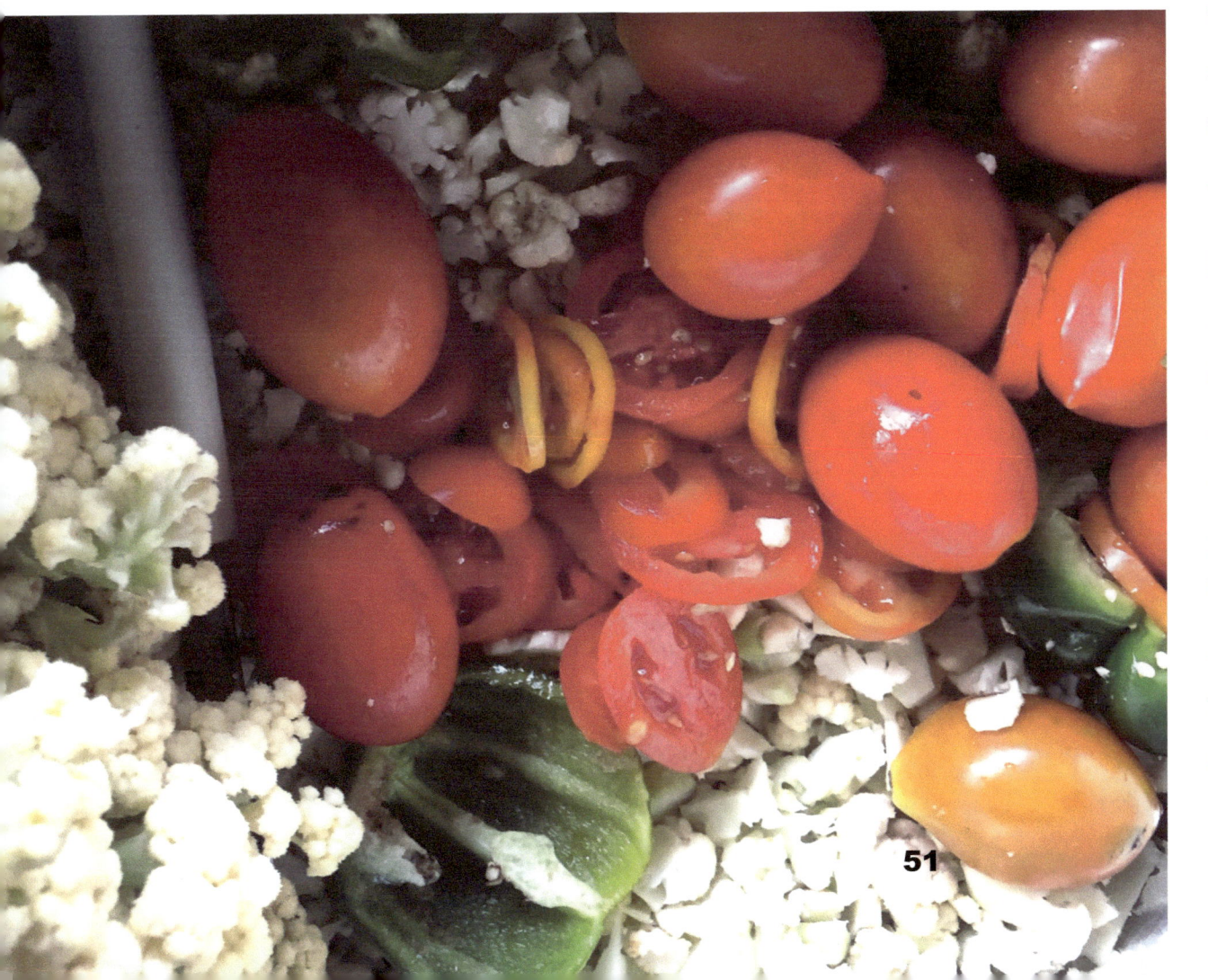

Celery

Celery is high in calcium, sodium, magnesium, manganese, chlorine, iron and iodine. It also contains vitamins B_1, B_2, B_3 and C, chlorine, silicon, phosphorus and potassium. It has a calming effect on the nervous system and is good for the blood, lungs and bronchial system. Celery has been recommended in treating diseases of the kidney, arthritis, rheumatism, neuritis, constipation, asthma, high blood pressure, excess mucous production, inflammation of the gums and loosening of teeth (pyorrhea), diabetes, brain fatigue, acidosis, gallstones, obesity, tuberculosis, anemia and insomnia. Because of its iodine content, celery serves as an excellent seasoning with other vegetables, nuts, seeds and grains.

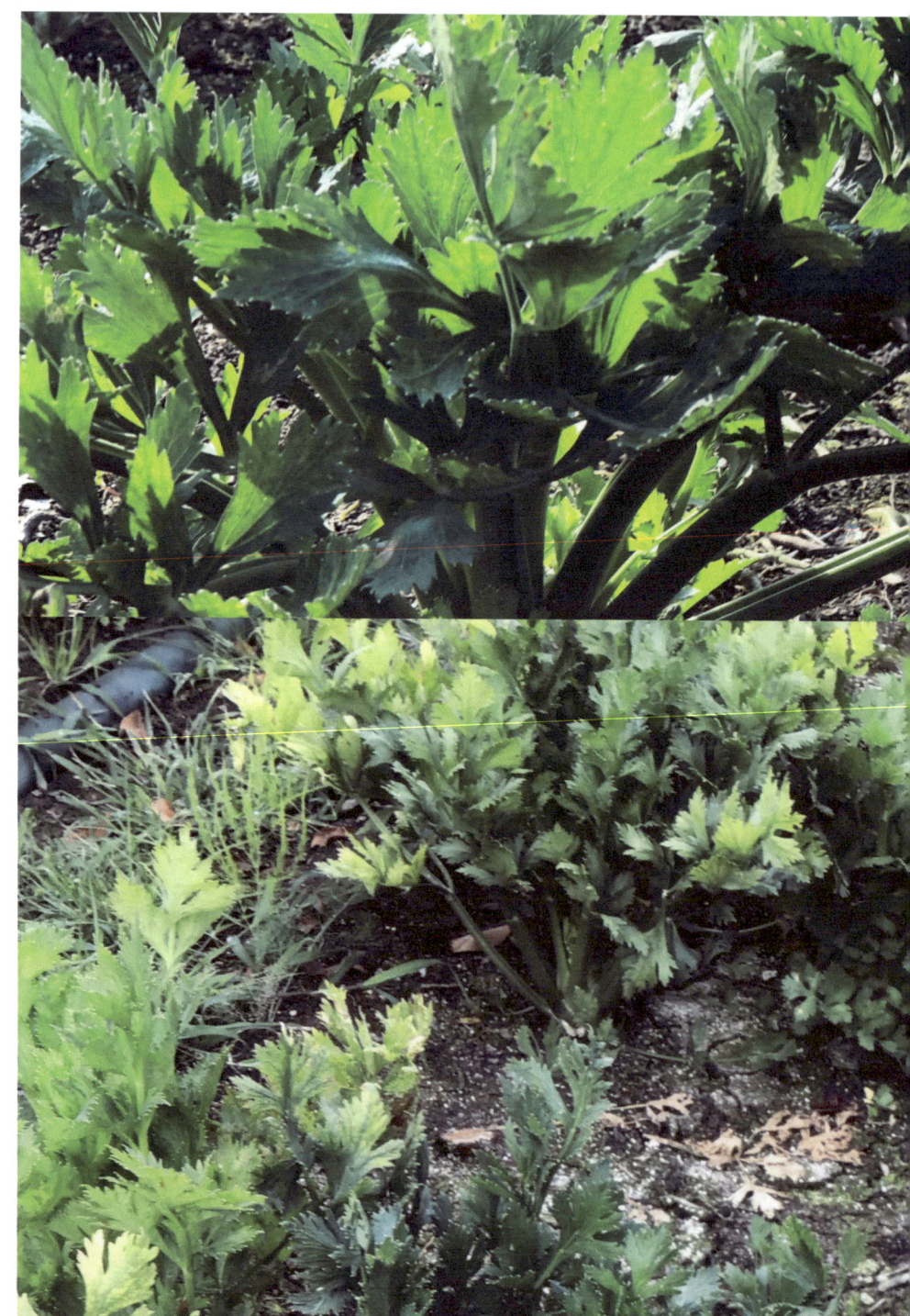

CHAPTER 5: BACK TO THE BASICS

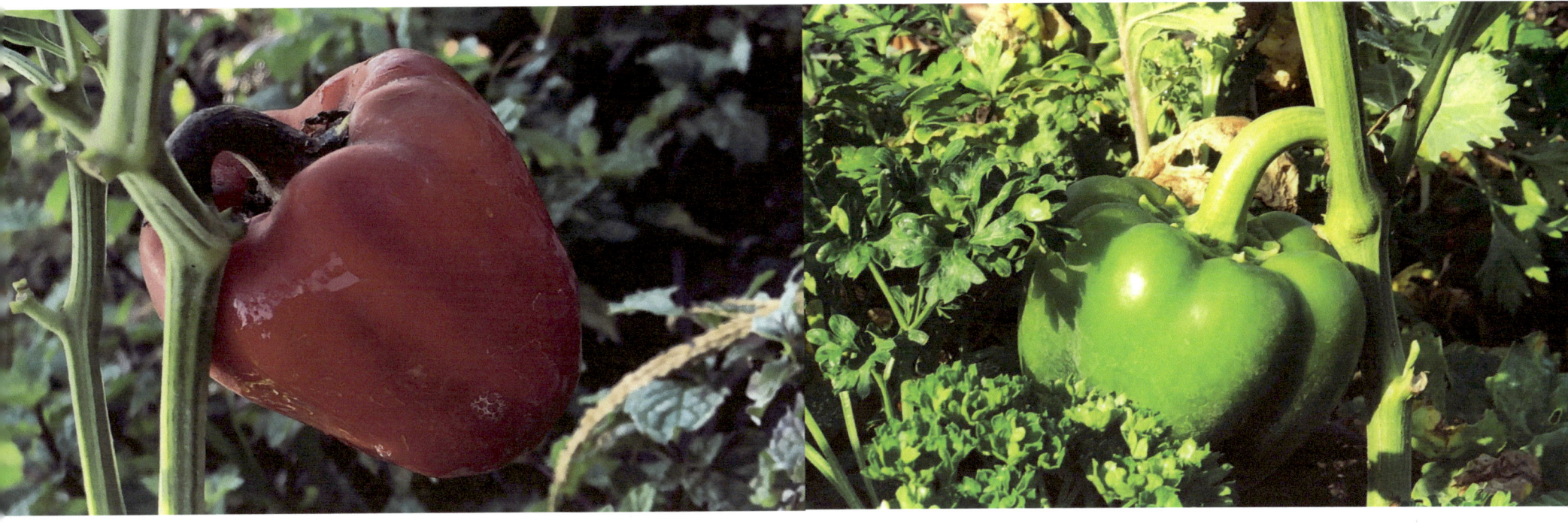

Bell Peppers

Peppers are fruits. They are a good source of vitamin C, potassium and silicon. Peppers also contain significant quantities of vitamins A, B_1, B_2 and B_3, calcium, iron, phosphorus and potassium. Red peppers are especially high in vitamin A and are an excellent source of vitamin B_6. Studies show that vitamin B_6 deficiency consistently impairs T-cell functioning in the immune system and results in a decrease in blood lymphocyte counts. Bell peppers are also recommended for liver disorders, obesity, constipation, gas, high blood pressure, improving circulation, toning and cleansing the arteries and heart muscle, and acidosis. Peppers are also good for the hair, nails and skin.

Garlic

Garlic surely provides some the world's most potent time-tested healing elements and its potent smell is what makes it so powerful. The active ingredient allicin turns into organosulfurs, which are the compounds that keep your cells safe from all the destructive cellular processes that can cause major chronic diseases. Garlic is a natural antiseptic; it helps prevent cancer, fights infection, and colds. Research also states that garlic may prevent or decrease chronic diseases associated with age, such as atherosclerosis, stroke, cancer, immune disorders, brain aging, cataracts, and arthritis.

Onion and garlic are said to keep evil spirits away and I believe it is true. Because anytime I eat garlic, all of the people with a superficial, artificial and unnatural frame of thought tend to run away

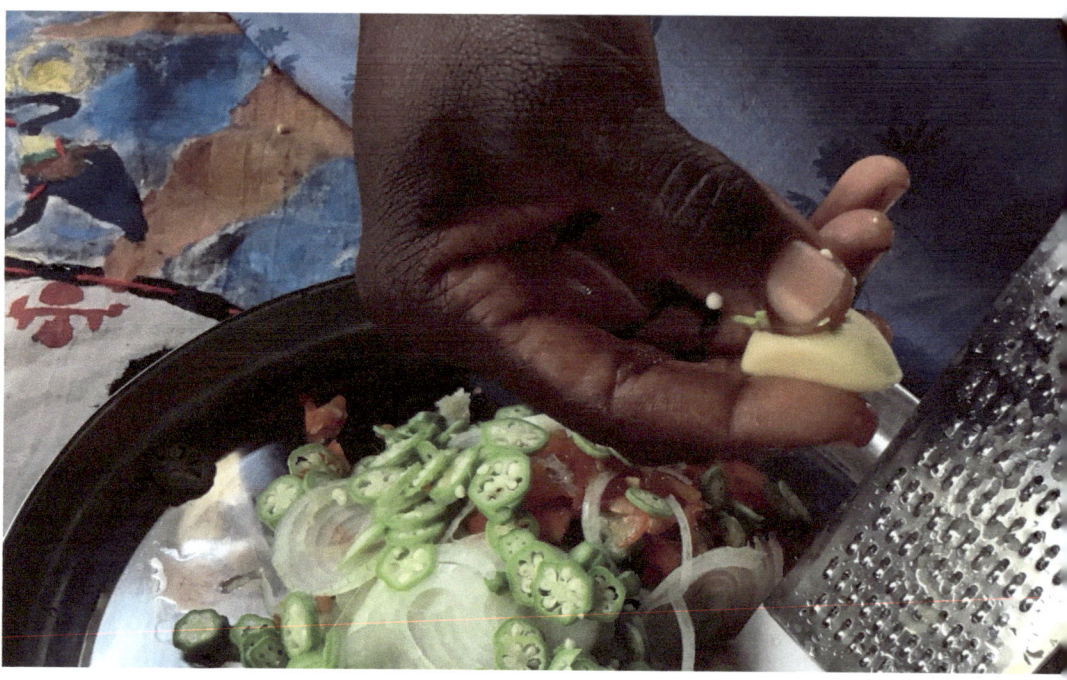

from me and they are definitely the evil spirits of the planet. Keeping the evil spirits away is notable enough; however, garlic has an extra potent ability to cleanse the blood and the body system, helping to eliminate toxins and waste from the body also making it good for the lymph. The lymph work as a part of the immune system to filter out harmful substances.

CHAPTER 5: BACK TO THE BASICS

Onion

Onions are a good source of sulfur and potassium. They also contain calcium, chlorine, selenium, phosphorus, iron, inositol, vitamins A, B_1, B_2, B_3 and C. Onions are diuretics, laxatives and good antiseptics. They help to drain mucous from the sinuses and cavities and loosen phlegm. Onions are good for the hair, nails and eyes, because of their sulfur content. They are recommended in cases of asthma, bronchitis, pneumonia, influenza, colds and tuberculosis.

Onions are also helpful in treating cases of low blood pressure, insomnia, neuritis, and vertigo. Because of their antiseptic properties, they can be used to destroy worms and parasites. Onion can be made into a poultice and applied to the chest to treat cases of inflammation of the lungs and applied directly to the skin to treat boils.

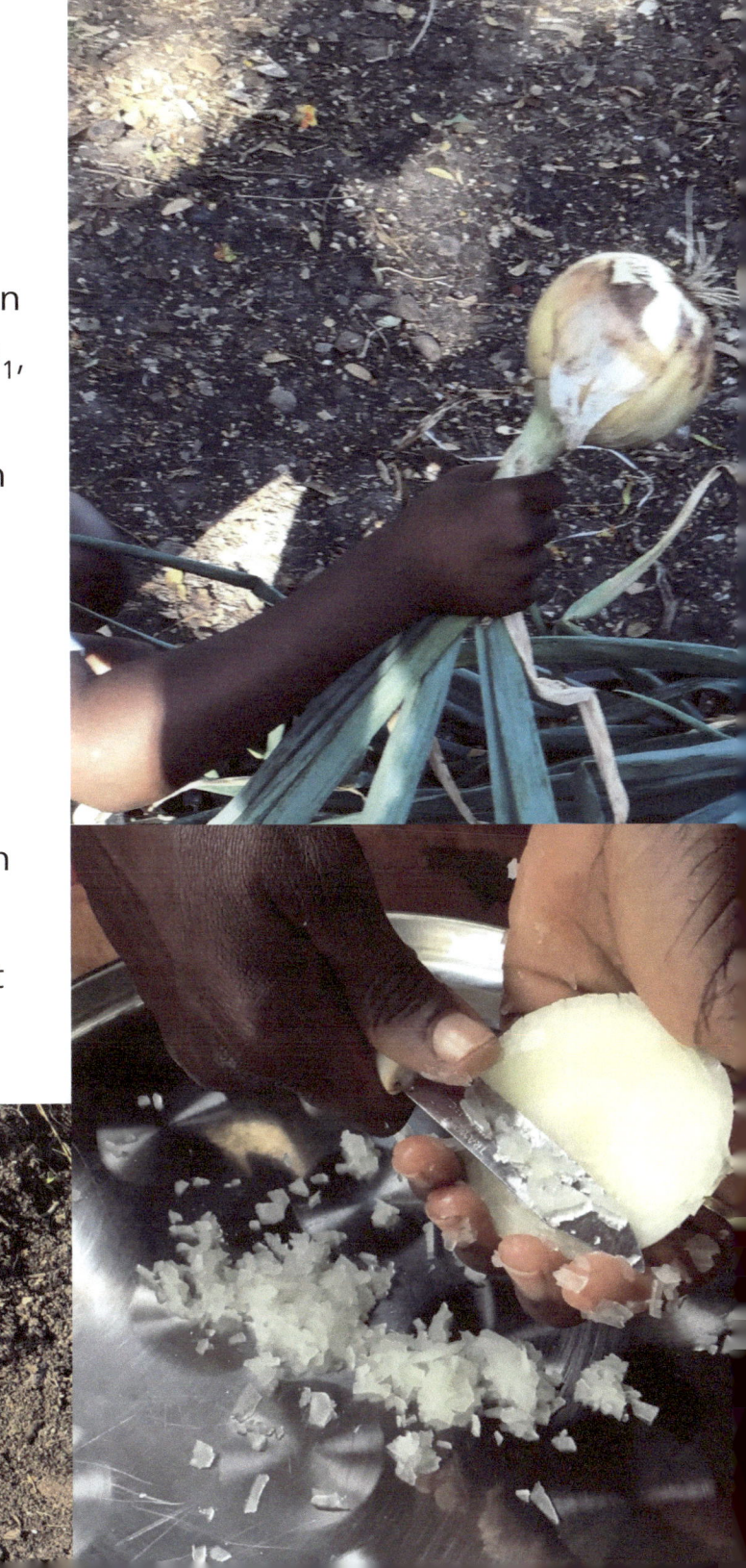

CODE GREEN: HIDDEN POWERS OF THE GARDEN TARGETING THE IMMUNE SYSTEM

Limes

Lemons and limes are best known for their antiseptic properties and can be used internally and externally for this purpose. From our experience, lime is one of the best antiseptics in the world, followed closely by its cousin, the lemon. We use lime juice as a main activating ingredient in our recipes. We use sliced lime or lemon and their juices, applying them directly to cuts, acne sores, boils and other skin sores. We have applied lime to insect bites, especially mosquito bites and other irritations for cleansing or relieving itching. While my family and I were living in West Africa, those in the neighboring villages often wondered why I and my family never came down with malaria. I'm sure that a contributing factor is the fact that as soon as one of us would get a mosquito bite, we would scrub the bite with lime. (I note that we also quickly consumed jungle bitter herbs for extra immune system protection). Lime juice can also be used

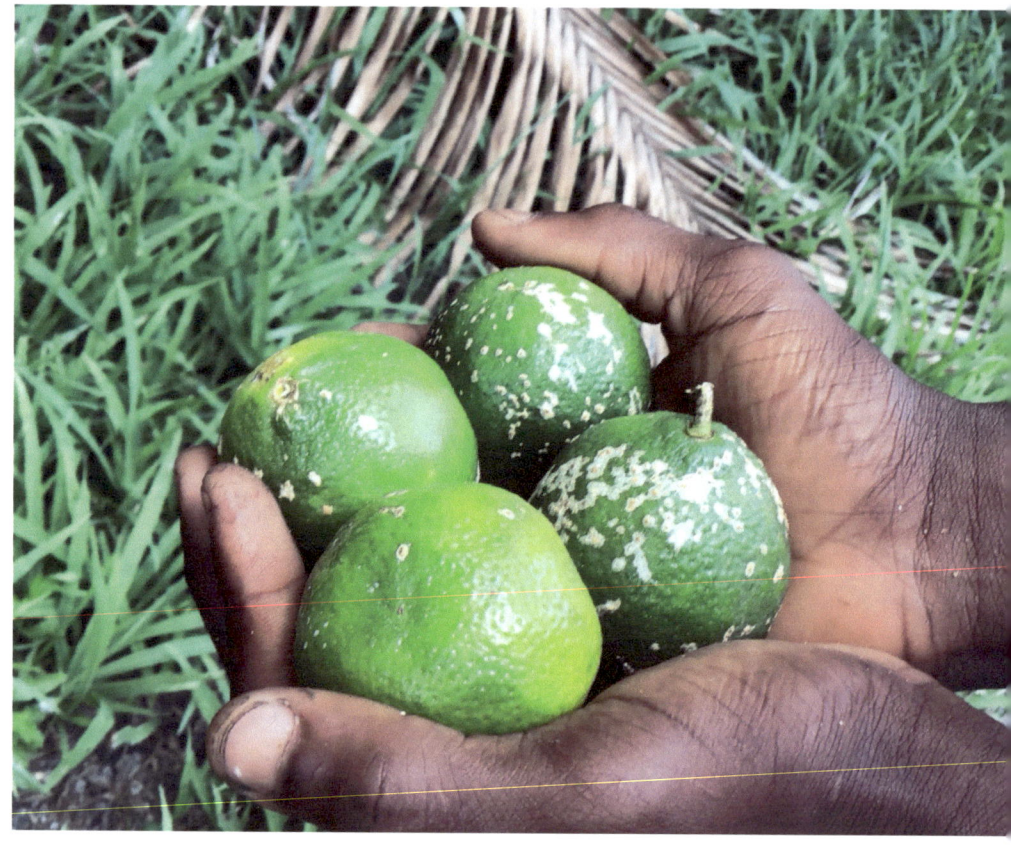

to relieve cold symptoms, such as cough and running nose. Limes also effectively treat the following conditions: rheumatism, arthritis, liver ailments, asthma, fever, pneumonia and neuritis. So, lime is definitely a superfoods antiseptic.

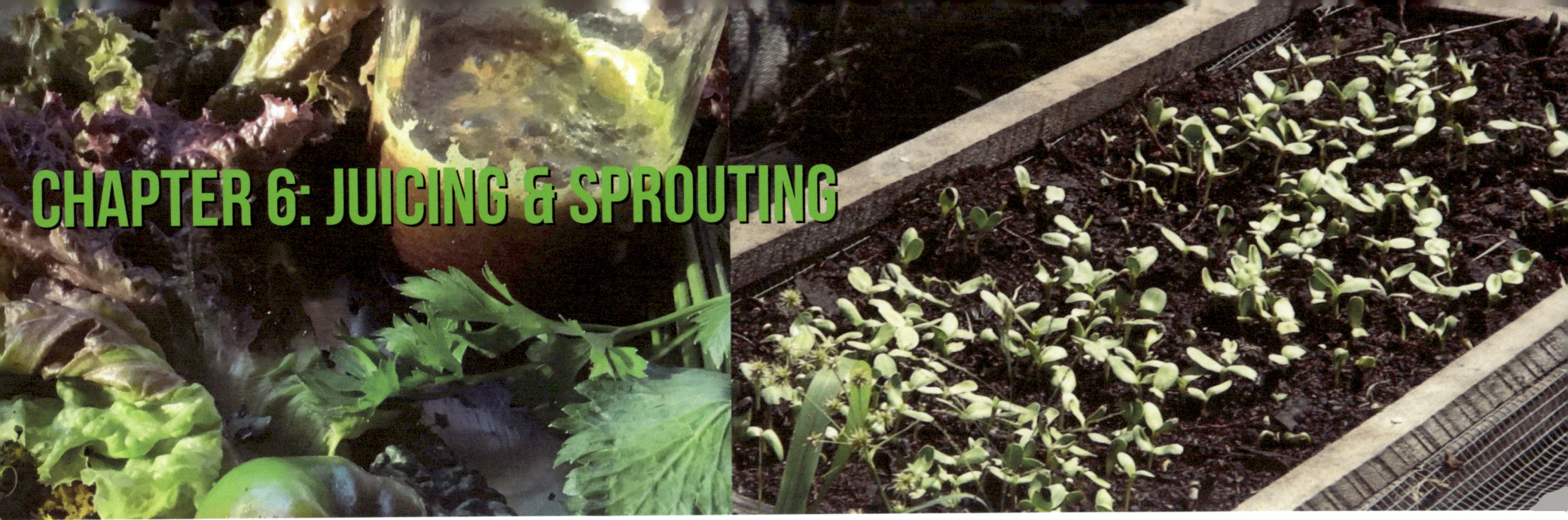

CHAPTER 6: JUICING & SPROUTING

Our mission in this chapter is to deal with the most expedient method of assimilating whole foods into the body. When we say assimilate into the body, I hope that everyone understands that the body has a special river that flows from the tip top of the head to the bottom of the toe. That river is called the blood/circulatory system which delivers oxygen, nutrients and biochemical messengers throughout the body. Therefore, it should be very clear that under any dire emergency, the quicker we can get whole, live, life enzymes into the bloodstream, the quicker we will be able to address any problem that the body may have in cleansing and/or healing itself. In other words, this red river of life is key to fueling a healthy immune defense system.

Juicing

When consuming live fruits, vegetables, seeds, nuts and grains, the most expedient way of getting those whole foods into the body with the least amount of tax on the body is through whole and live juicing. When I say juicing, it is extremely important to recognize that we are talking about extracting every drop of liquid content from the particular fruit or vegetable so as to formulate a live and wholesome food that we call juice. In order to do that, one must use the proper kind of juice extracting mechanism.

The ideal situation is to take a press that has no relationship with heat whatsoever and to have the juices extracted through the use of pressure. This kind of cold-pressing extraction provides an effective way to obtain whole and complete nourishment from the juicing process without excess oxidation. After obtaining the proper kind of extraction mechanism, you are now on the road to a completely unique experience in whole health.

Looking at it as such, one must comprehend that there is one kind of nutritional support for cleansing and another for building and repairing the whole body system. The live foods for cleansing, basic and simple, are fresh fruits.

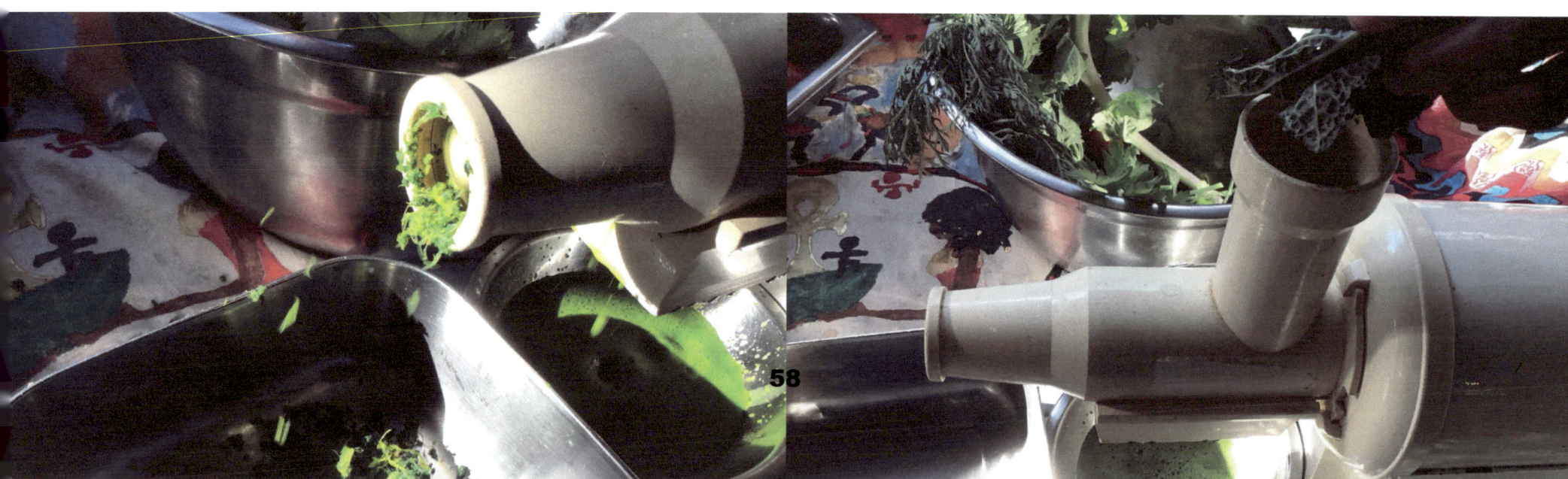

CHAPTER 6: JUICING & SPROUTING

Kwatamani First Genesis Tribe live foods approach is to view all foods as holistic living healing sources for the body, the brain and the spirit.

Fresh, live, whole, organic fruits. The live foods for repairing are just as simple, fresh vegetables. Fresh, live, whole, organic vegetables.

When we want this cleansing and repairing healing process to take place as quickly as possible, the best method to use is live juicing. Fresh, live, wholesome, organic juicing. Drinking water regularly also helps to flush out toxins from the body, supporting the immune system in efficient functioning. This is another way to encourage a healthy immune defense system. However, juicing adds essential nutrients for building, repairing and strengthening the immune system.

We included some juices and juice combinations that are very popular with the I in I, juices that I'm sure will greatly assist you in your holistic living mental, physical and spiritual development.

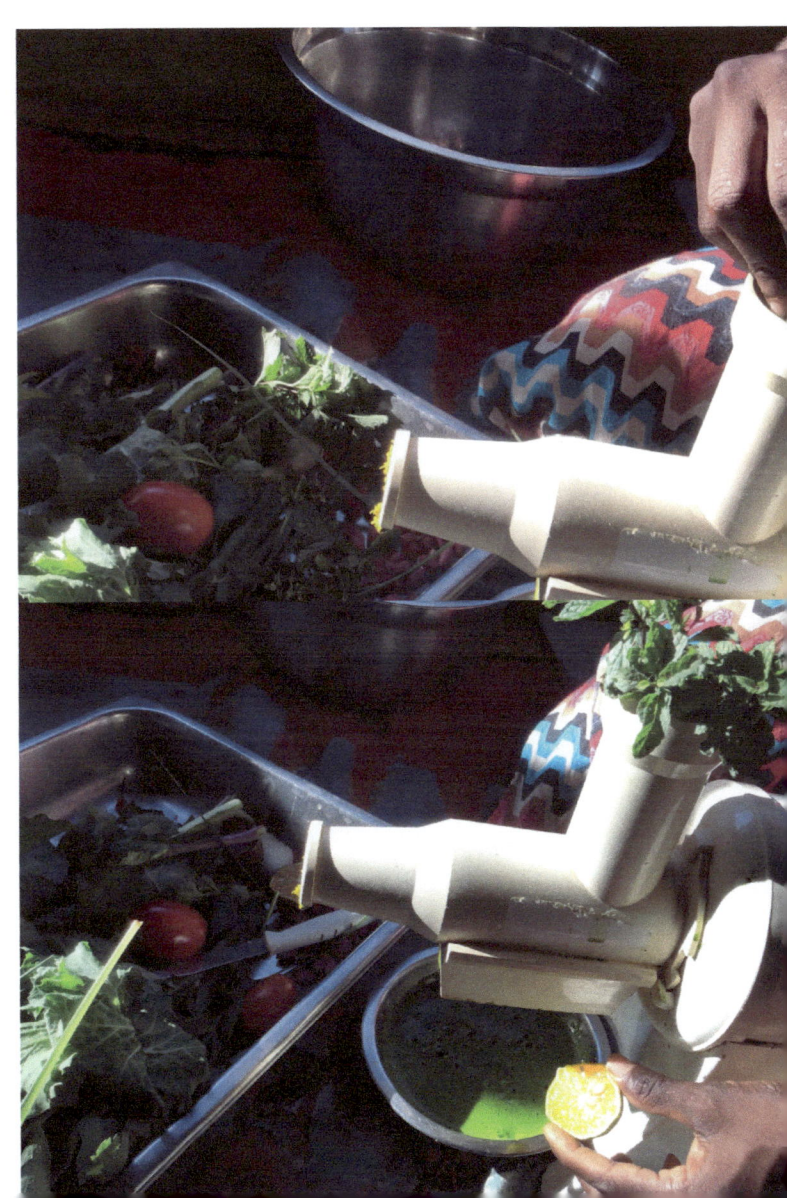

59

CODE GREEN: HIDDEN POWERS OF THE GARDEN TARGETING THE IMMUNE SYSTEM

Juicing Preparation and Instructions

A variety of fresh organic/veganic greens are a potent, nutrient-rich tonic to support all of the body systems with special attention to the vitamins, minerals and antioxidants that provide optimum fuel to strengthen the immune defense system.

Washing tip

For greens with a firm, hard fiber stem, cut or pick the leaves off the stems. For greens and other vegetables with a tender stem, there is no need to remove the stem. Get a big bowl of water to wash the handful of leaves that you picked and any other vegetables. Squeeze a little lime juice, or use a cap full of raw apple-cider vinegar in the water as an antiseptic cleanser.

Swish the leaves around and shake off excess water. Rinse the leaves two more times in clean water (purified or spring) to remove any additional dirt particles. Then push the greens and other vegetables through your juicer. This juice is packed with super supreme greens and loads of vitamin A, iron, calcium and other minerals. A wonderful tonic for the teeth, bones, blood and eyes.

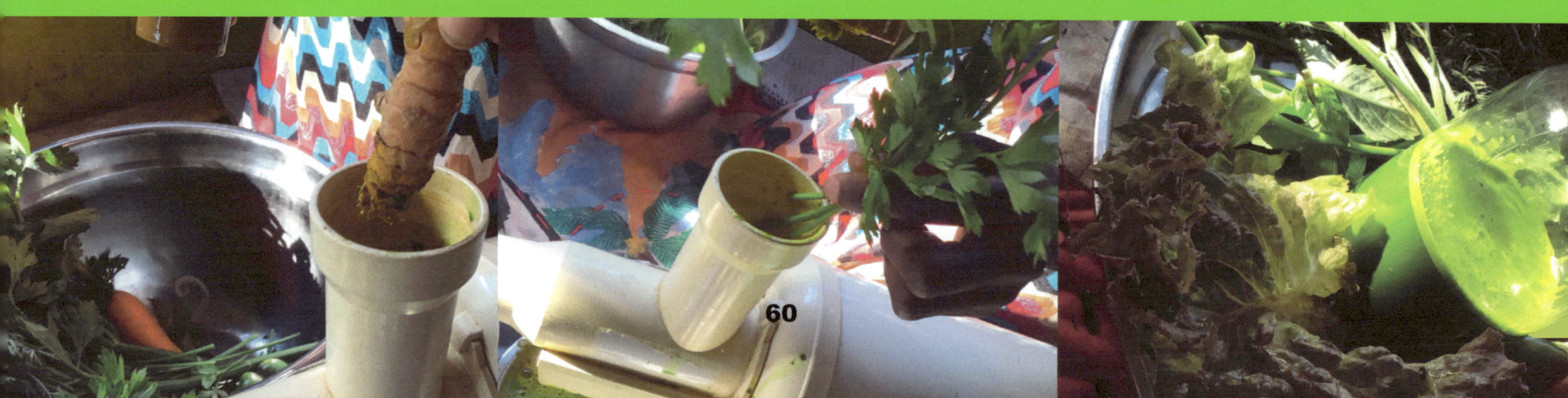

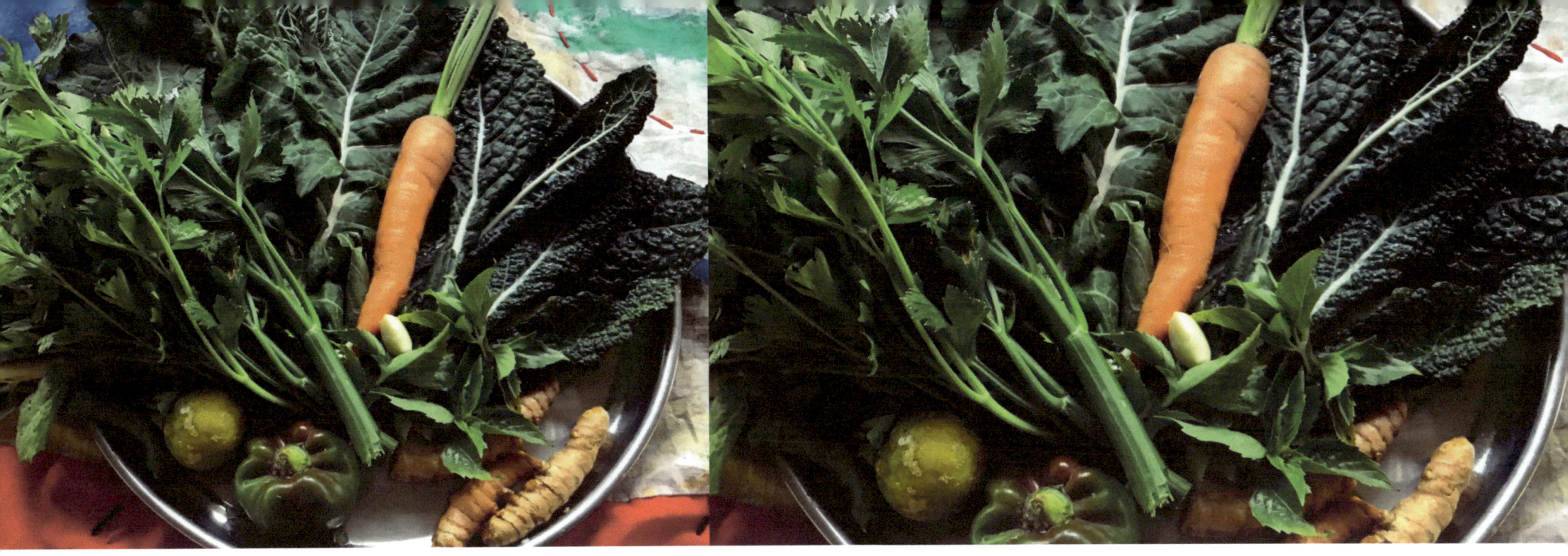

Go Green Immunity Tonic

kale

collard greens

celery

parsley

basil

garlic

carrot

turmeric

green bell pepper

twist of lime

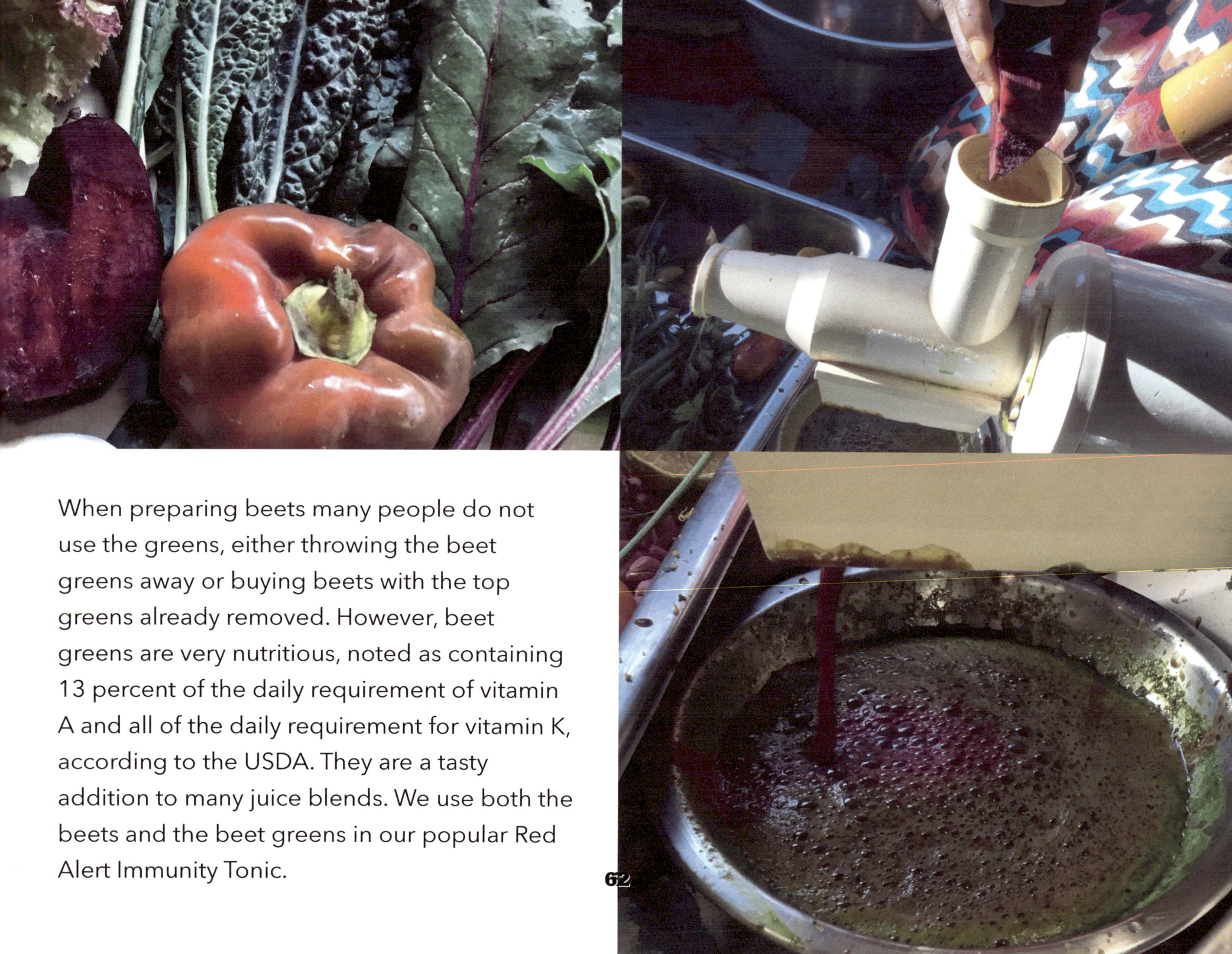

When preparing beets many people do not use the greens, either throwing the beet greens away or buying beets with the top greens already removed. However, beet greens are very nutritious, noted as containing 13 percent of the daily requirement of vitamin A and all of the daily requirement for vitamin K, according to the USDA. They are a tasty addition to many juice blends. We use both the beets and the beet greens in our popular Red Alert Immunity Tonic.

CHAPTER 6: JUICING & SPROUTING

Red Alert Immunity Tonic

tomato

kale

red beets

red beet greens

fire red lettuce

red bell pepper

small piece of garlic

small piece of onion

mint

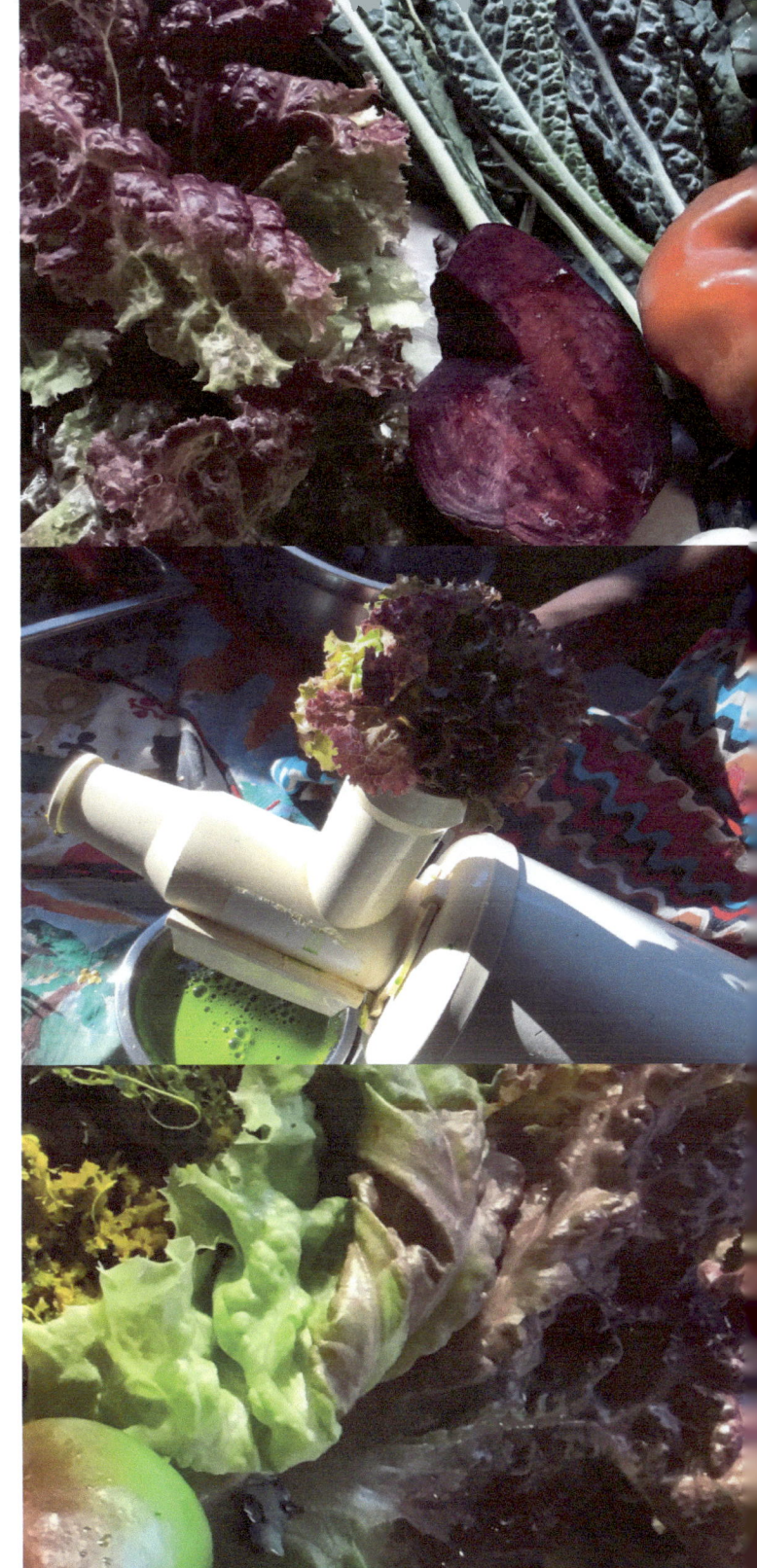

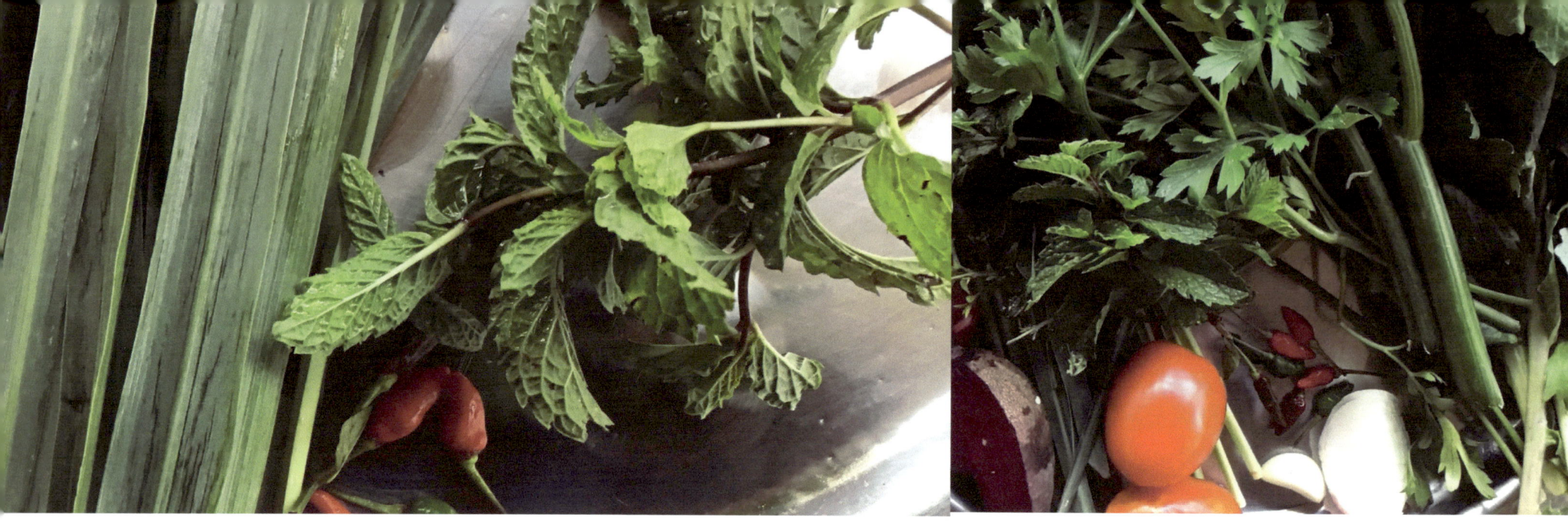

Immuno-Green Super Soup

combination of leafy green vegetables

tomato

celery

beets and beet greens

garlic

mint

parsley

lemon grass

peanuts, handful

African Bird peppers, to taste

twist of lime

pinch of evaporated sea-water salt

CHAPTER 6: JUICING & SPROUTING

Super Soup Instructions

When I was younger and addressing the consumption of fresh vegetables, people often suggested we go to a restaurant and order soup and salad. That is to say, boiled food substances and a small bowl of pale lettuce on the side. I have to say, this had no appeal to my holistic living appetite so I decided to take it a step further. Here is the recipe for one of our very popular Kwatamani Super Soups, a high-powered immune system enhancement soup. Put this together and be prepared for a very wholesome soup that will stimulate your taste buds and quickly activate the natural and innate response of body enzymes to gain full nutritional benefits.

Place all vegetables, peanuts, herbs and African Bird pepper in the blender. Add quarter onion and one garlic. Blend until smooth. Pour mixture into a separate bowl. Add a pinch of sun evaporated sea water to taste. Add fresh-squeezed lime juice to taste. Stir well and enjoy. You can add diced tender vegetables if you prefer a chunky-style soup.

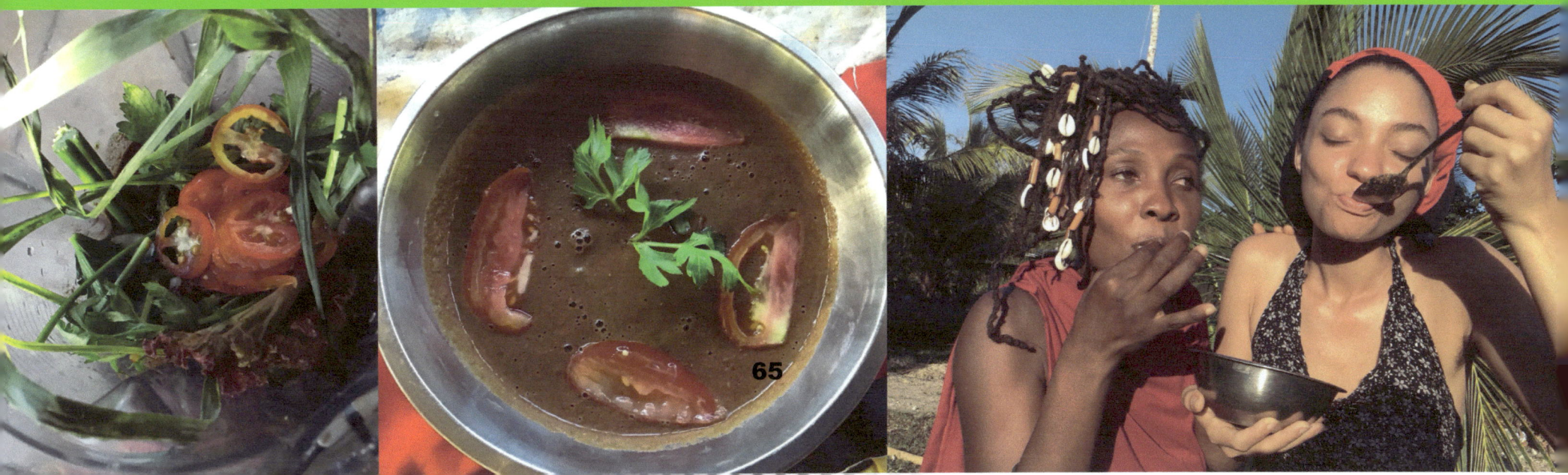

CODE GREEN: HIDDEN POWERS OF THE GARDEN TARGETING THE IMMUNE SYSTEM

Sprouting seeds is an easy way to grow your own food. You can sprout indoors and you don't need a lot of space. You can safely store an amount of seeds and then sprout them when needed. You can sprout almost any legume, seed or nut. From sunflower seeds to lentils to chickpeas. Grains, nuts and beans are all seeds. Each seed contains vitamins, minerals, proteins, fats and carbohydrates in storage, waiting for the necessary conditions to begin growing. You can sprout many kinds of seeds, There are commonly eaten seed such a sunflower seeds and pumpkin seeds. Sprouting involves soaking seeds, nuts, legumes or grains for several hours, then repeatedly rinsing them until the begin to develop a root.

Different seeds require different amounts of water when soaking, but a basic rule is three parts water to one part seed. You can determine how much seeds you want to sprout at one time. Keep in mind that once the seeds soak and begin to grow the amount of sprouts will be much more than the original amount of seeds.

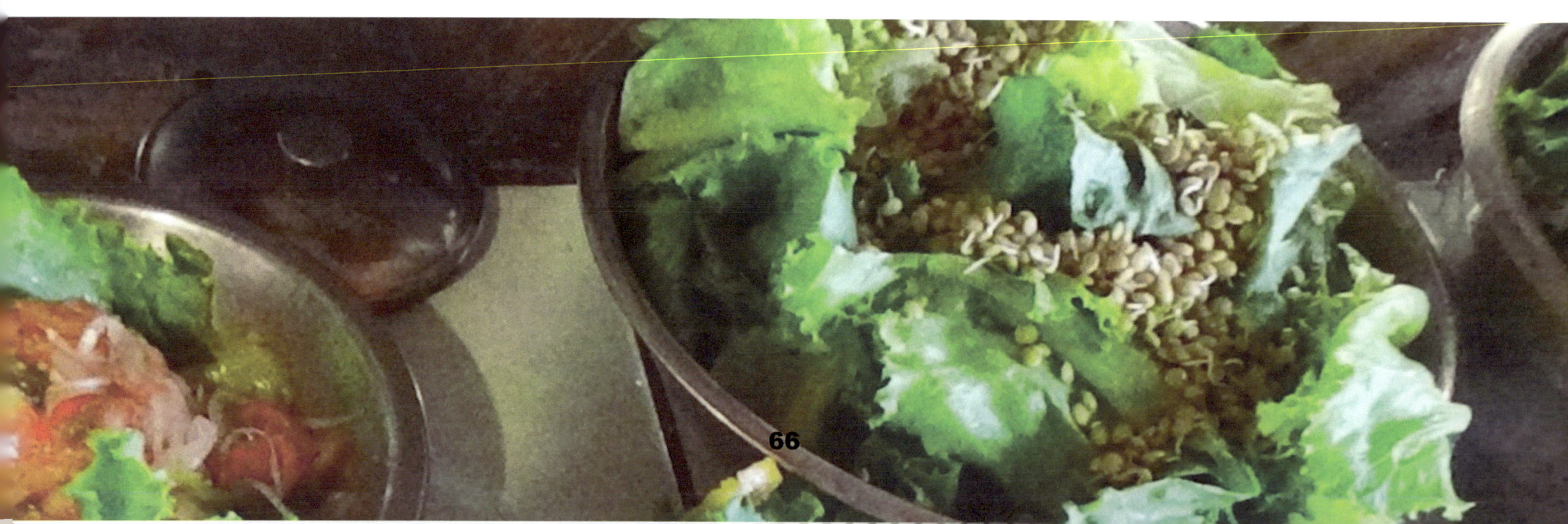

CHAPTER 6: JUICING & SPROUTING

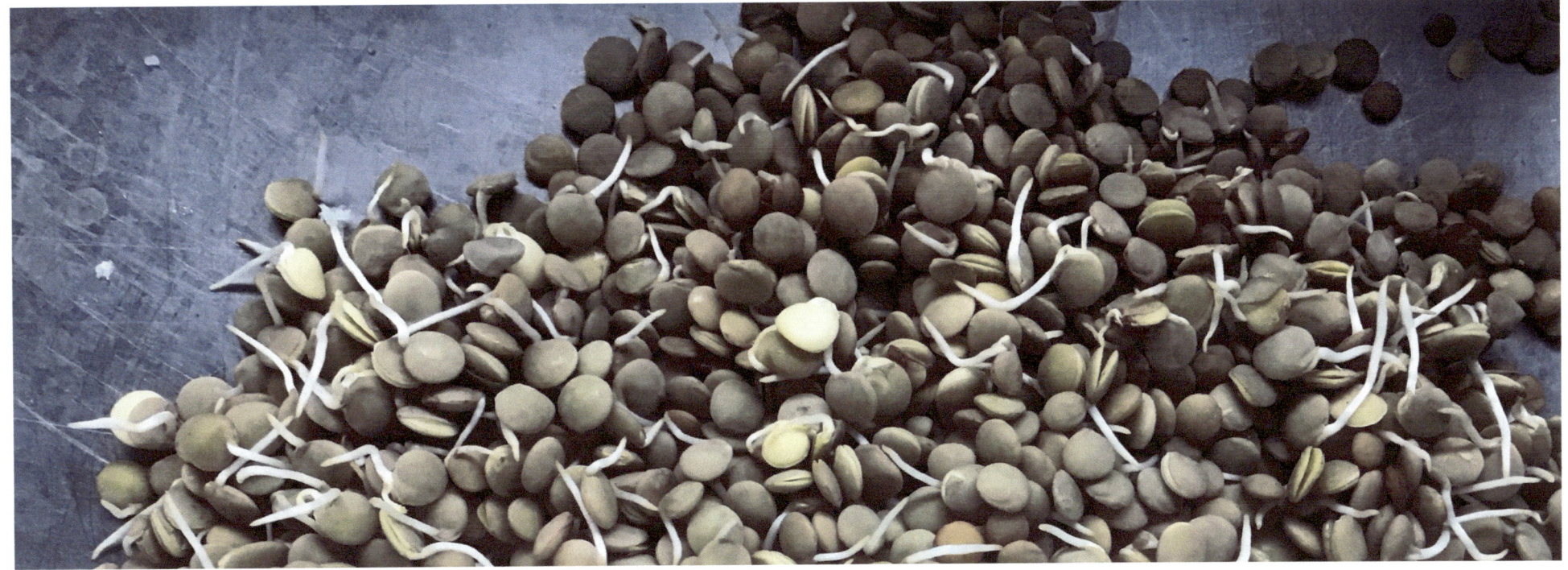

You will need to make sure that the sprouts are able to drain well and receive enough air circulation.

When the seed begins to sprout, a tremendous flow of energy is released and natural chemical changes occur.

▶Enzymes are activated which are necessary for food ingestion.

▶Proteins are converted into amino acids, the basic buiding blocks of every living cell.

▶Starches change to simple sugars.

▶Minerals combine for increased absorption.

▶Vitamin content increase from three to 12 or more times.

▶Chlorophyll and carotene content increase dramatically when exposed to sunlight.

Sprouts offer many health benefits. They are a rich source of antioxidants, making them very beneficial for the immune system.

▶ Soak seeds overnight (6 to 12 hours) in water. You can use a bowl or a glass jar. The optimal time for soaking is between 8 and 10 hours.

▶ Rinse seeds 2 to 3 times daily, allow them to drain, either in a tilted bowl or jar.

▶ Sprouts are ready to eat within 2 to 4 days, when the sprouts are about 1/4 inch.

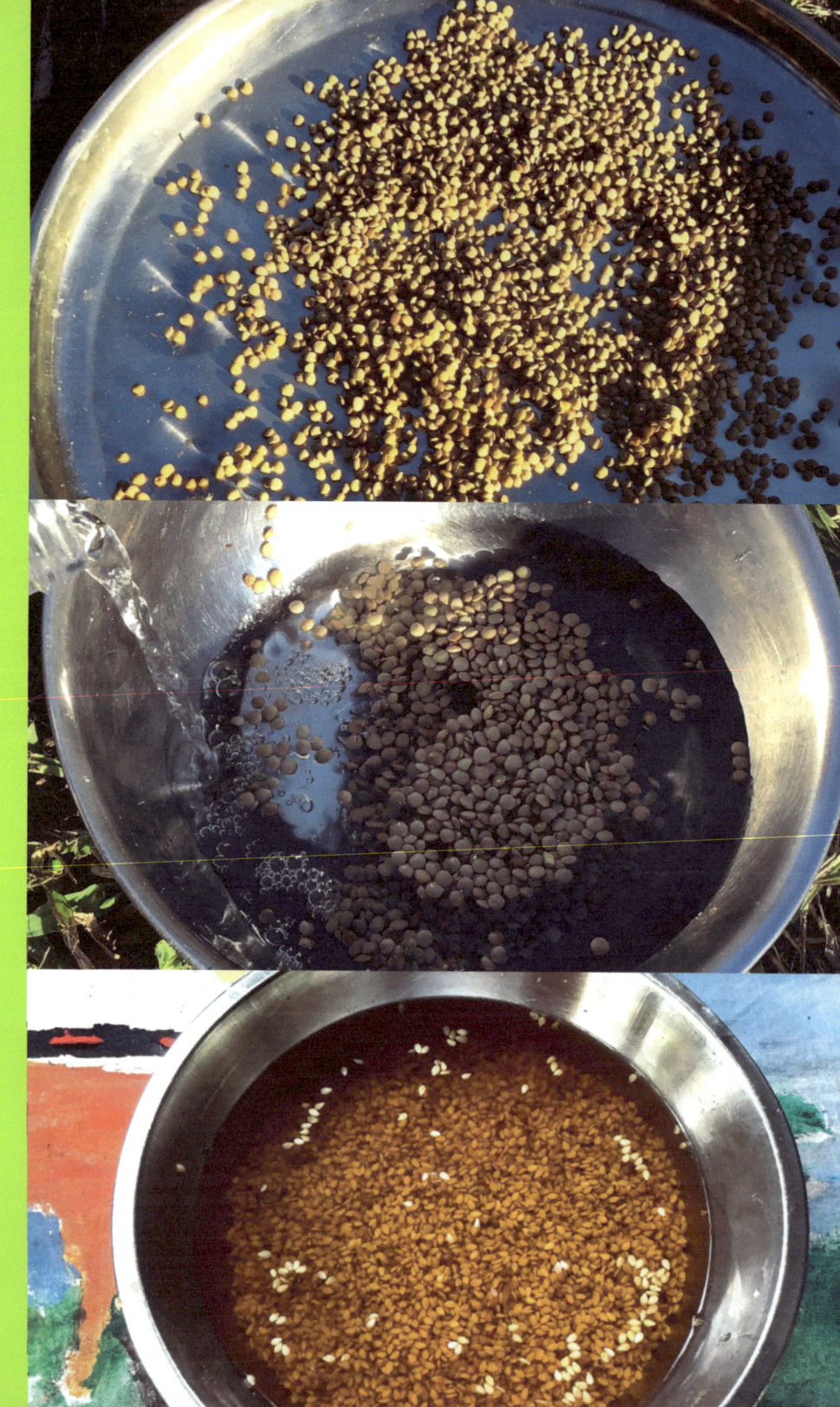

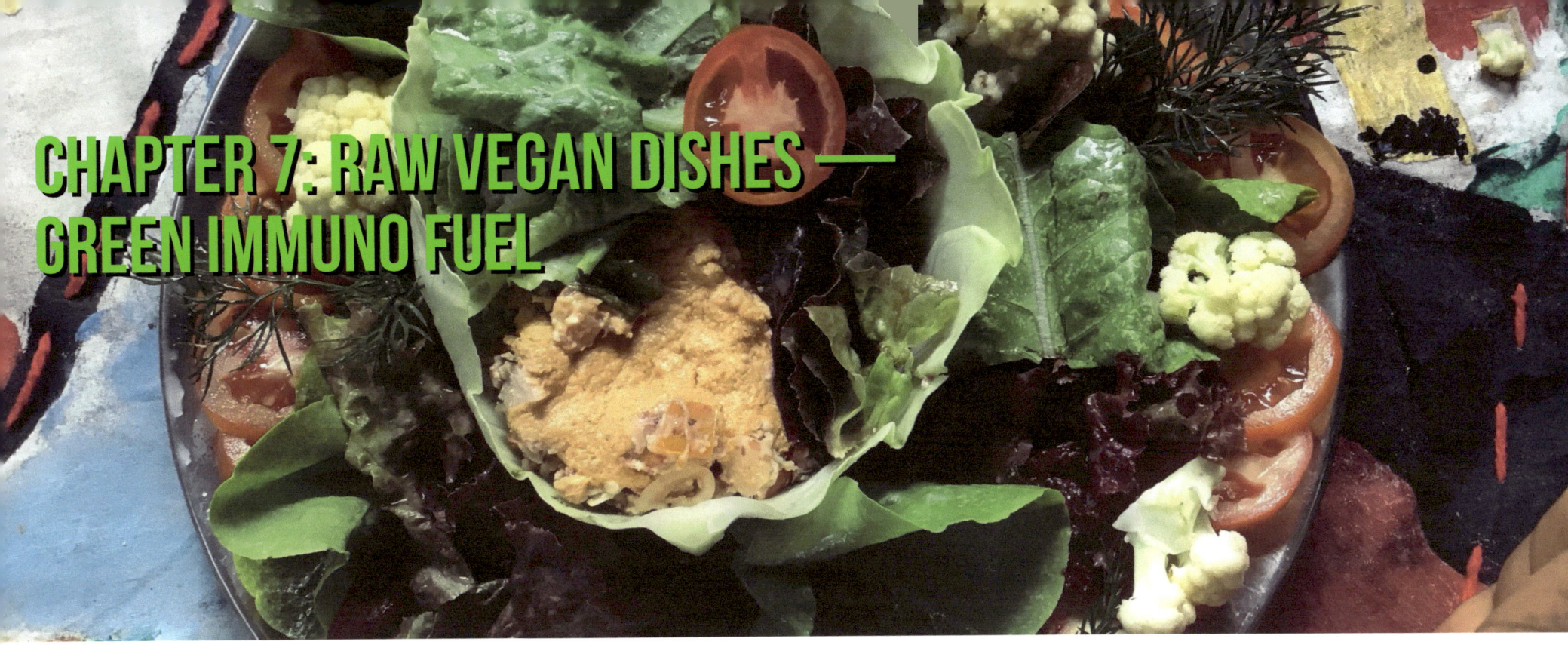

CHAPTER 7: RAW VEGAN DISHES — GREEN IMMUNO FUEL

We have explored some of the basic elements of raw and living fruits, vegetables, seeds and nuts which have been scientifically identified and classically accepted as needed by the body. We further identified the divine foods of the trees of life which definitely have these elements. It is also a known factor and must be clarified at this point in time that there are thousands of trace elements that have not even been identified yet, trace elements that can only be found in live foods.

No matter how much time scientists spend in the lab for centuries to come, it will still equate to the fact that no part or sum of parts is greater than its whole. That is to say that the life element of food and the life element of the body requires whole and live active enzyme relationships in order to be completely wholesome.

MARINATED MIXED GREENS

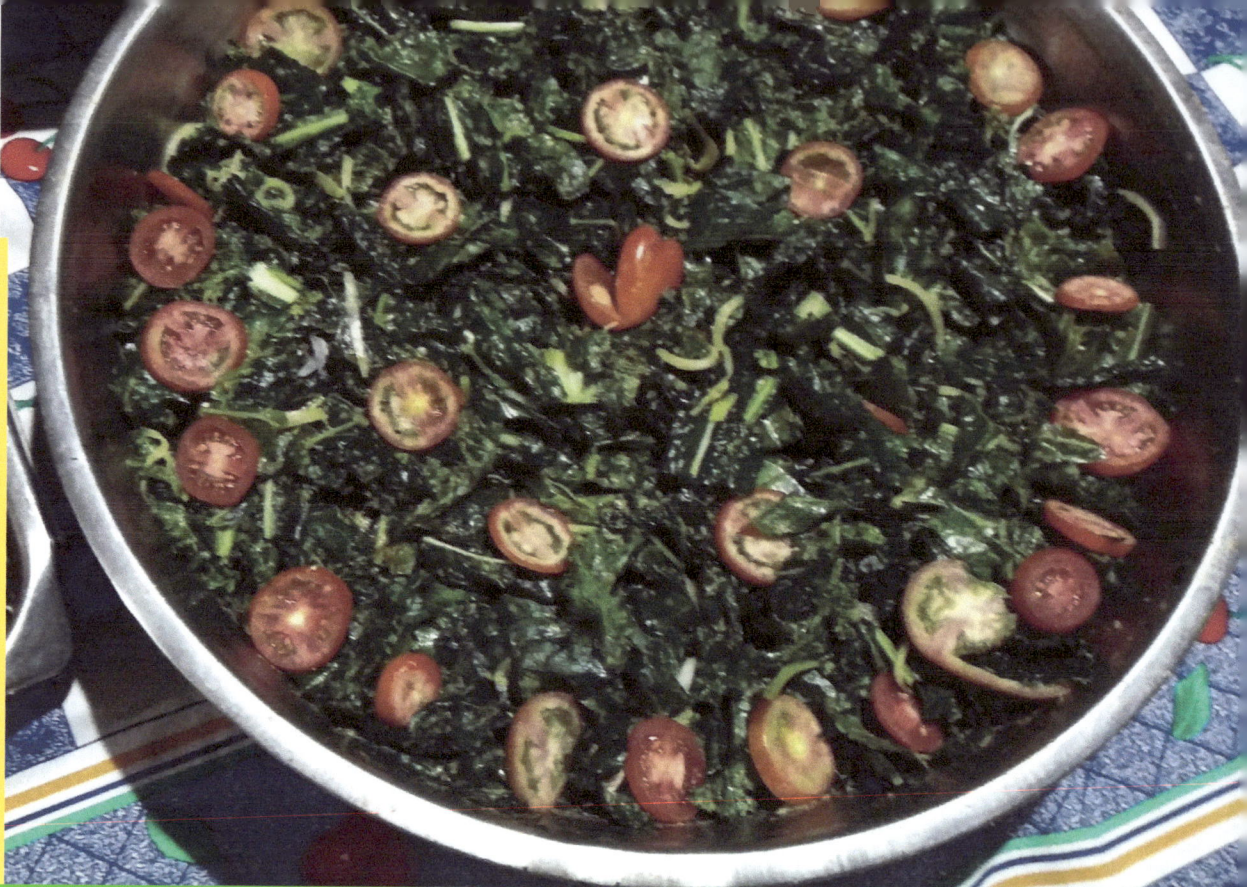

Ingredients

kale

greens, variety

tomato

sweet onion

lime

coconut oil

sun-evaporated sea water

Preparation Instructions

1. We urge that you give even greater attention to the handling and washing of those fruits and vegetables that you buy from a market or from any other source outside your home. In those cases, you do not know who has been handling your produce or what their hygienic patterns may be.

2. Finely slice the leafy greens and put in a large mixing bowl. The special cutting technique requires you to hold the greens firmly and shave across the top of the greens to get a thin shredding result.

3. Finely slice one tomato and one third sweet onion over the greens. Add one and a half teaspoons fresh-squeezed lime, one and a half teaspoons coconut oil, and a pinch of sun-evaporated sea water. Mix well and eat.

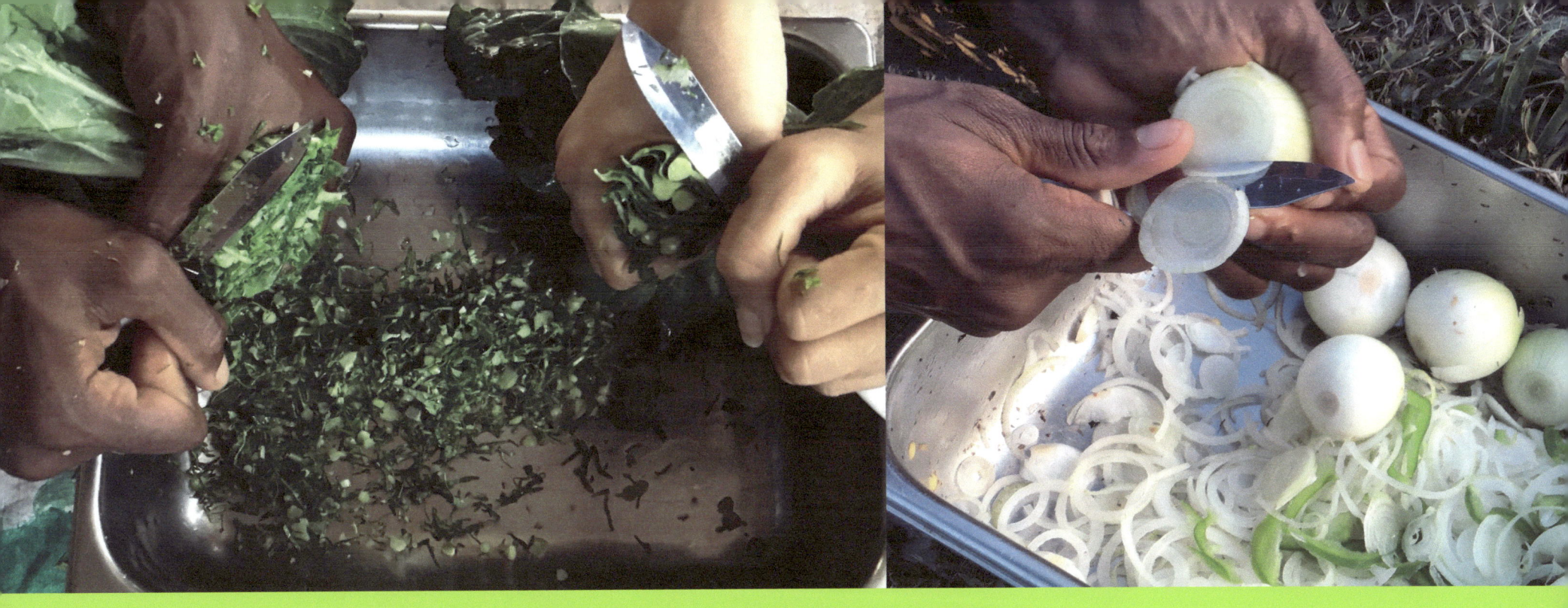

A most wonderful part of this recipe is that you can use so many different green leafy vegetables in this marinated mixed greens dish. Experiment with the varieties of kale, collard greens, arugula, and Chinese greens, such as bok choy and choy sum. The textures and flavors are sure to satisfy your taste buds while providing the full-nutrient impact of the greens.

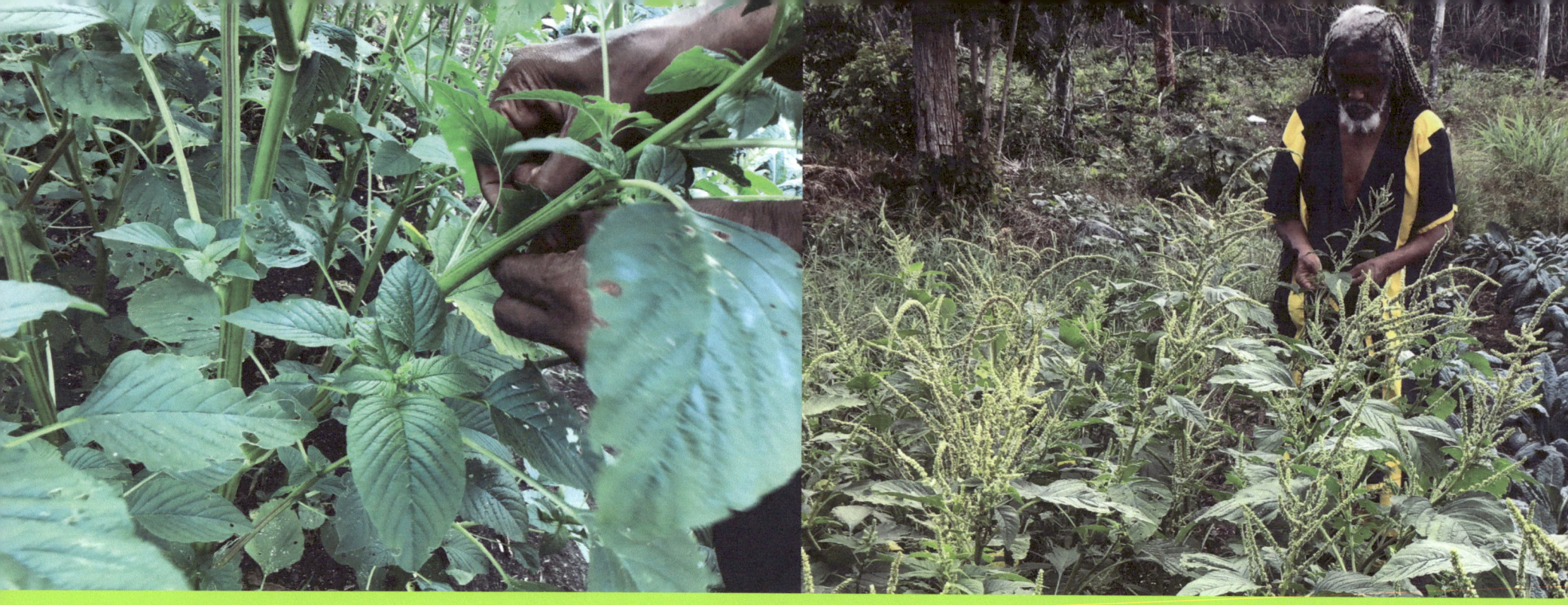

Popular Island Bush Greens: Callaloo

A favorite Caribbean vegetable, also known as green leaf amaranth, Indian or Chinese spinach, and shen choy, consumed in many traditional dishes. The young leaves and stems have a tender mild taste, similar to spinach, bok choy, collards, kale and Swiss chard, making Callaloo an excellent choice in many greens recipes.

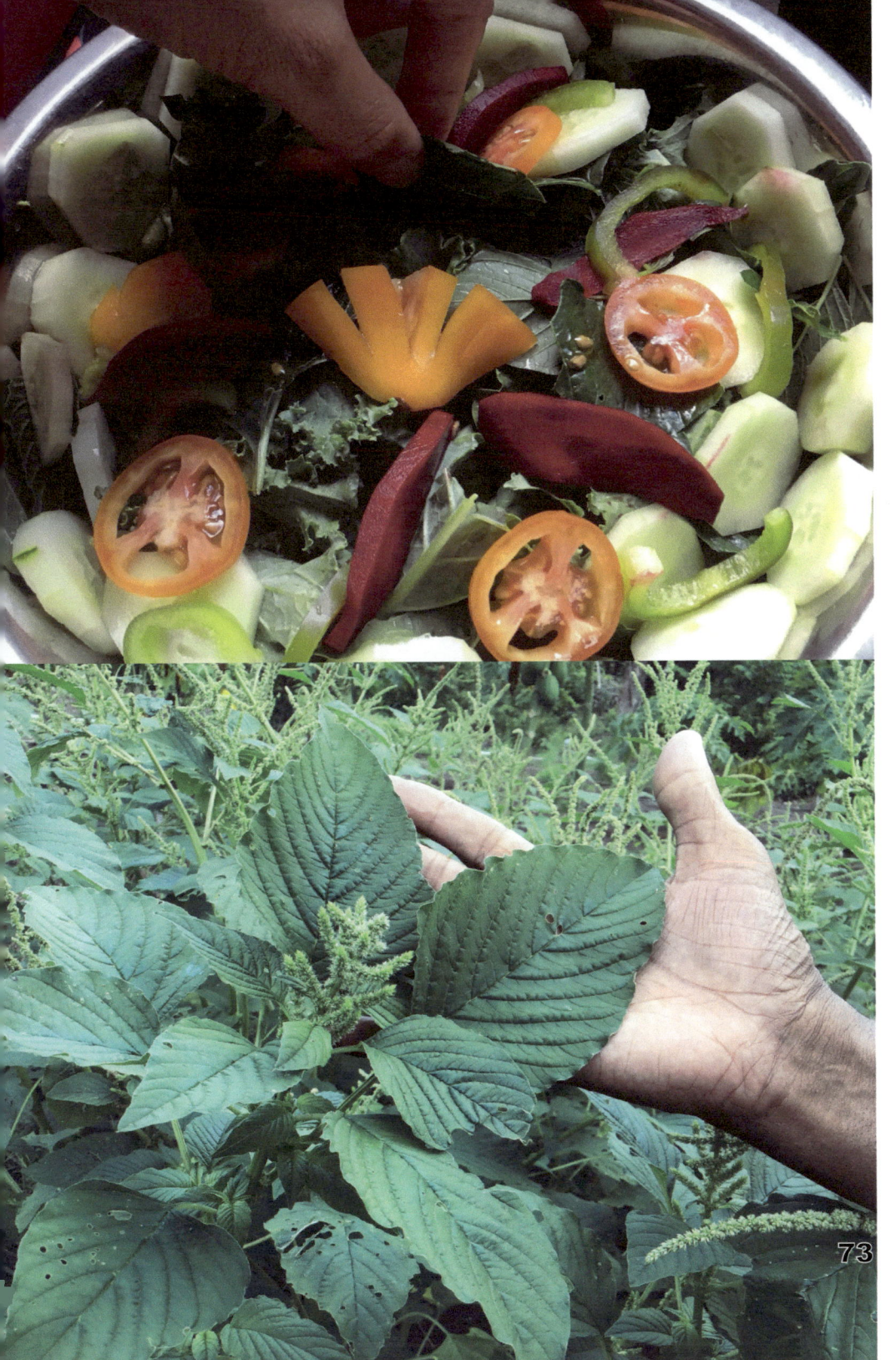

Callaloo Nutritional Benefits

The variety of callaloo Amaranthus viridis, better known as Chinese spinach or Indian kale, should not be confused with the callaloo foundin the eastern Caribbean, which refers to the leaves of the dasheen plant. It is noted that the leaf vegetable used in some regions may be locally called "callaloo" or "callaloo bush", originated in West Africa served in different variants across the Caribbean.

Callaloo, provides excellent nutritional support as a spinach-like green. The leaves are high in iron and calcium, vitamin C and K, super rich in antioxidants, protein, Omega 3 and 6. When preparing Callaloo and other greens, adding lime juice to the recipe enhances vitamin C to improve the absorption of iron into the body.

The immune system as a primary protective factor for the body is greatly enhanced by nutrient-rich fruits, vegetables, seeds and nuts.

SESAME SEED SUPREME

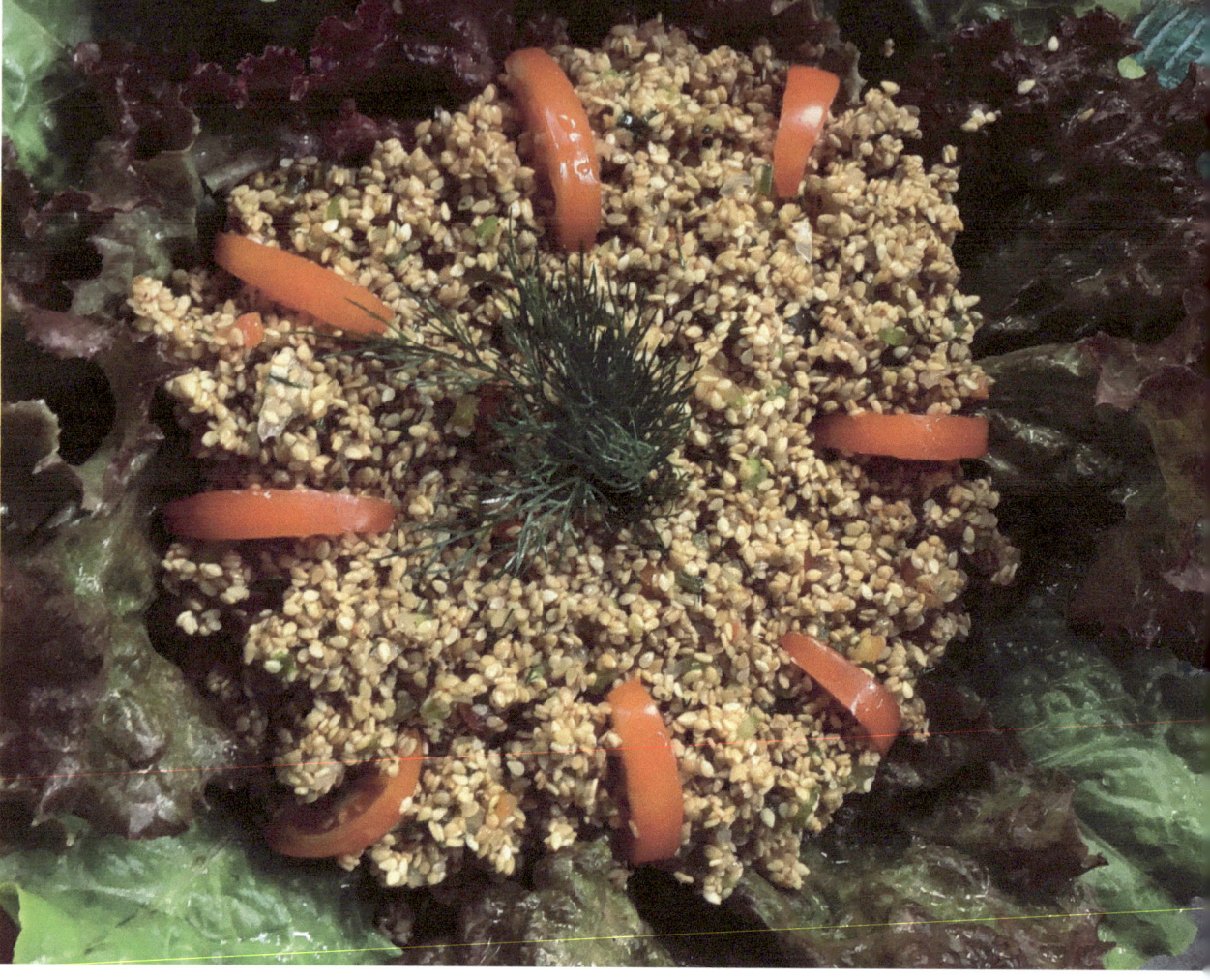

Ingredients

raw sesame seeds, unhulled onion

celery

bell pepper

tomato

garlic

dill

lime

coconut oil

sun-evaporated sea water

Sesame seeds are a good source of several nutrients that are important for immune system function, including zinc, selenium, copper, iron, vitamin B_6 and vitamin E. The body requires zinc to develop and activate certain white blood cells that recognize and help eliminate invading pathogens. These nutrients are also needed for blood cell formation and function. Sesame seeds are also good for the nerves, cellular function, metabolism, the heart and liver and for removing intestinal worms. Sesame seeds can be made into a sesame milk which the I in I have used to provide early nourishment during the children's weaning process.

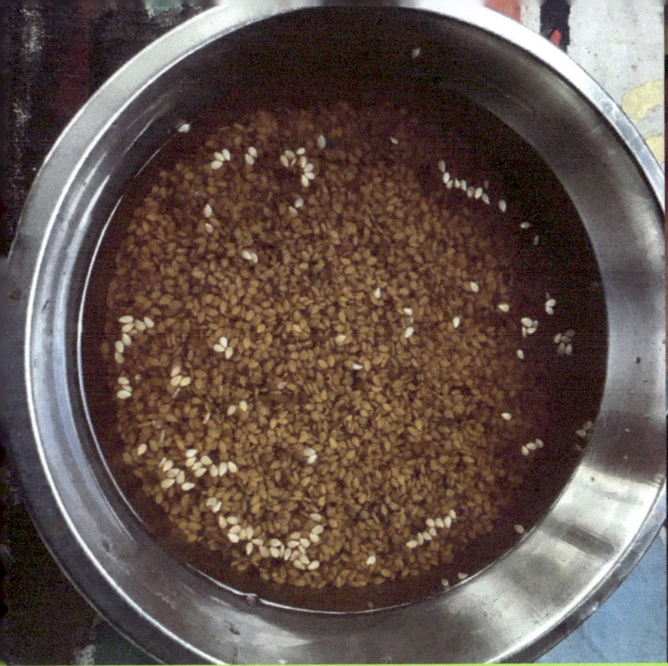

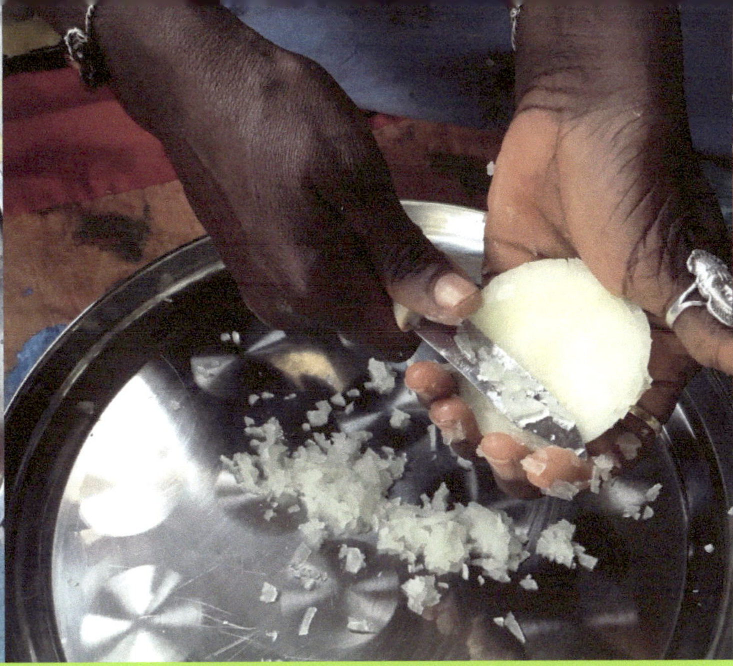

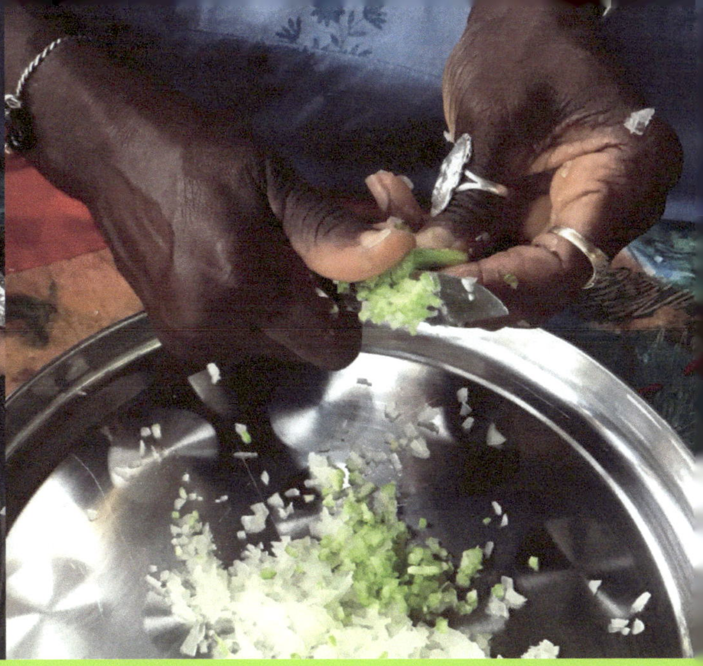

1. Rinse half of an 8-ounce cup sesame seeds and soak in spring water. Set to the side. Make sure you give your sesame seeds a few hours to soak in order to activate the seeds' wholesome nutritional factors.

2. Dice one half small onion, one third stalk celery, one small tomato, and a quarter bell pepper.

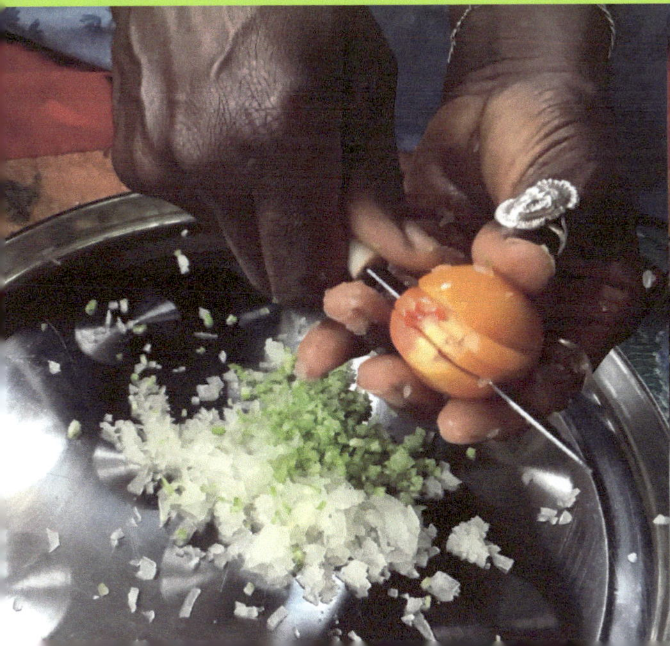

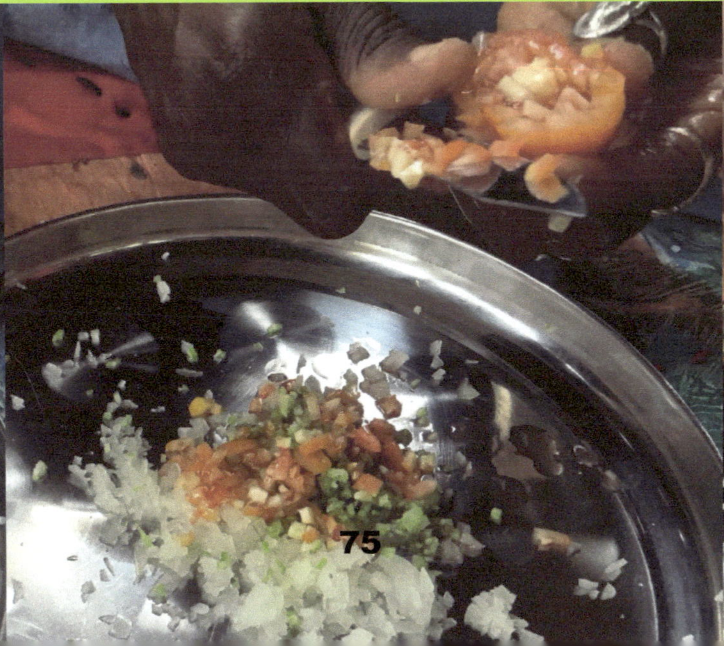

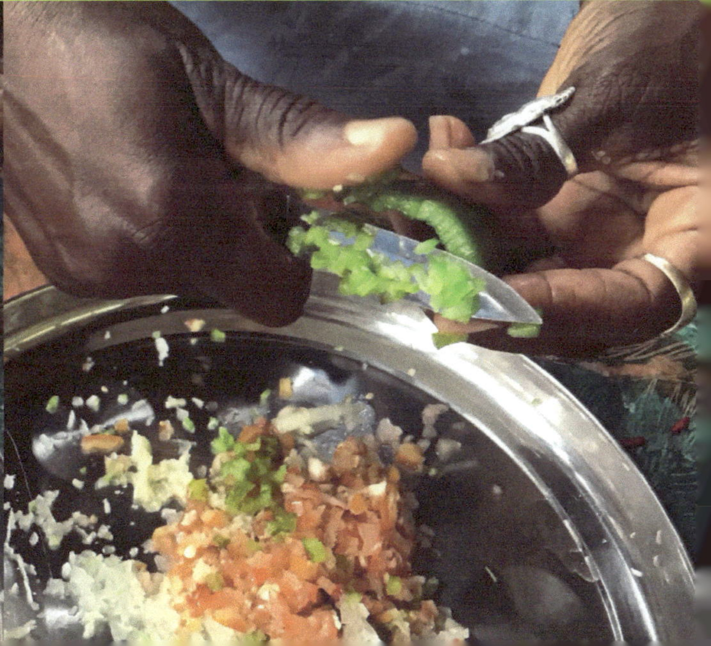

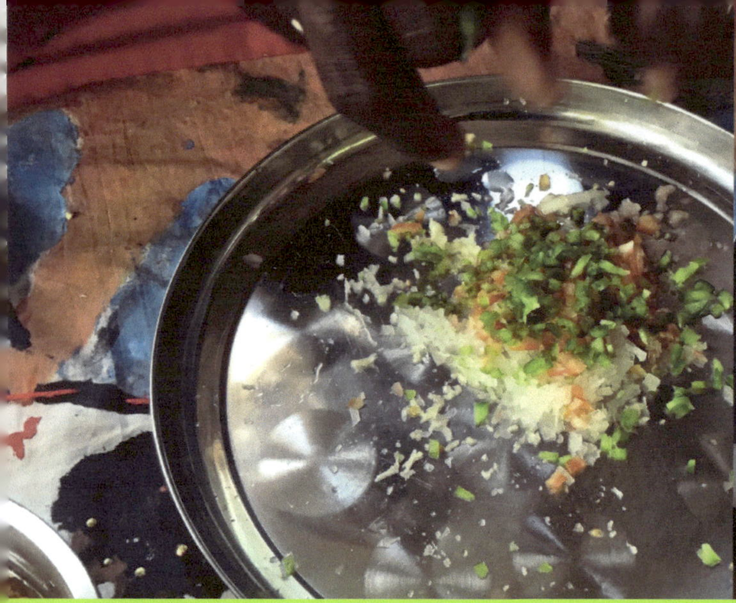

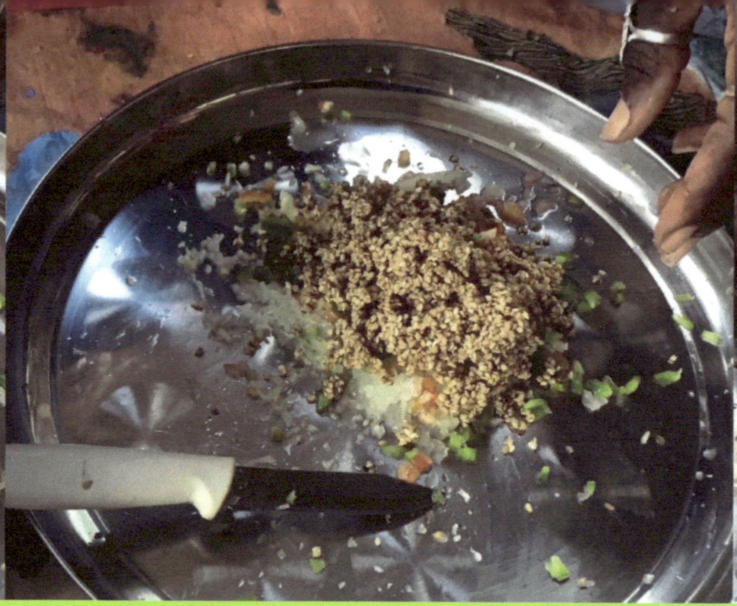

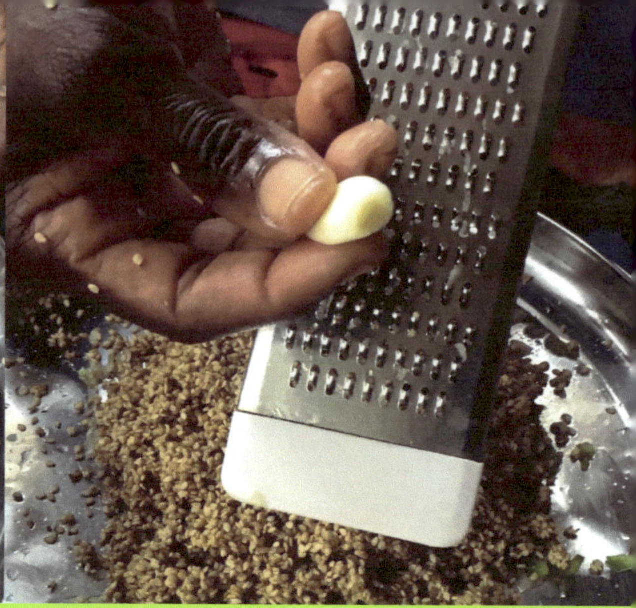

3. Put diced vegetables in a bowl.

4. Drain the water from seeds. Add sesame seeds to vegetables.

5. Add ½ clove pressed garlic and mince two stems of dill into the mixture.

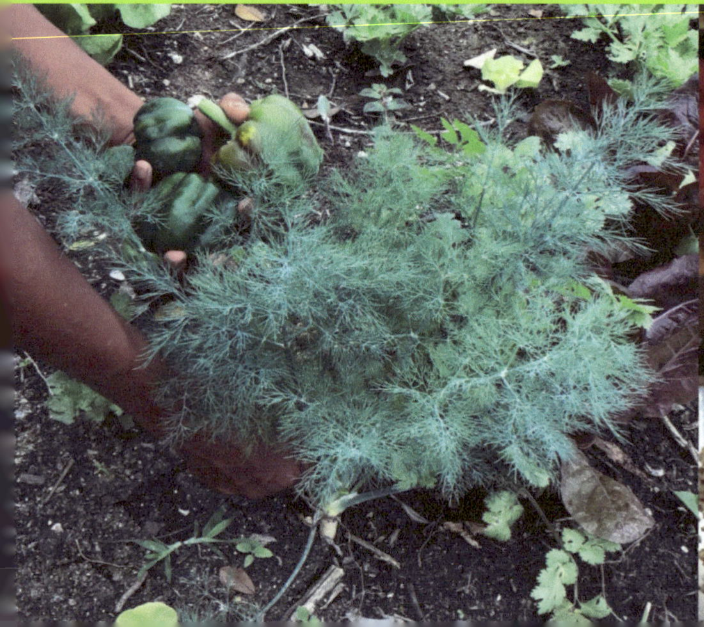

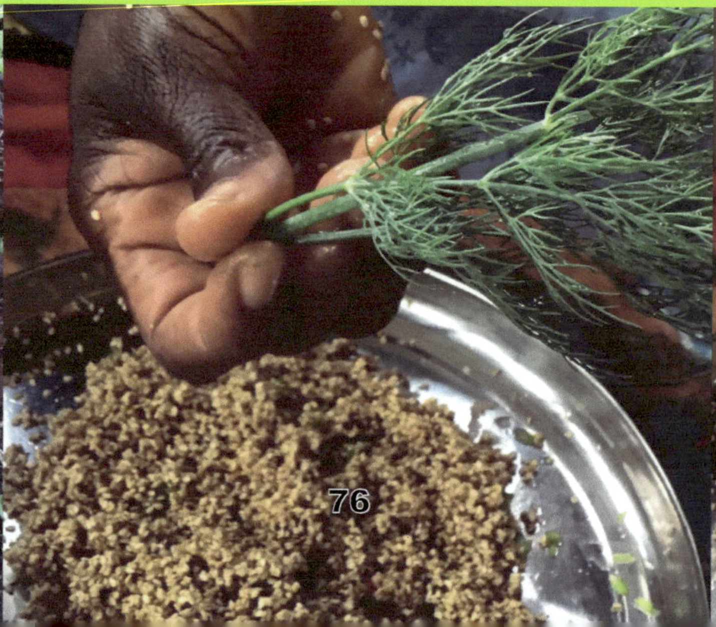

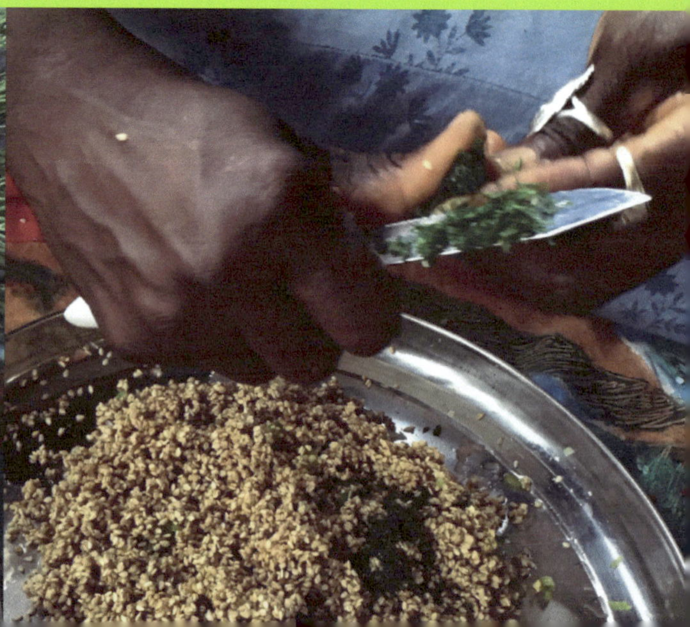

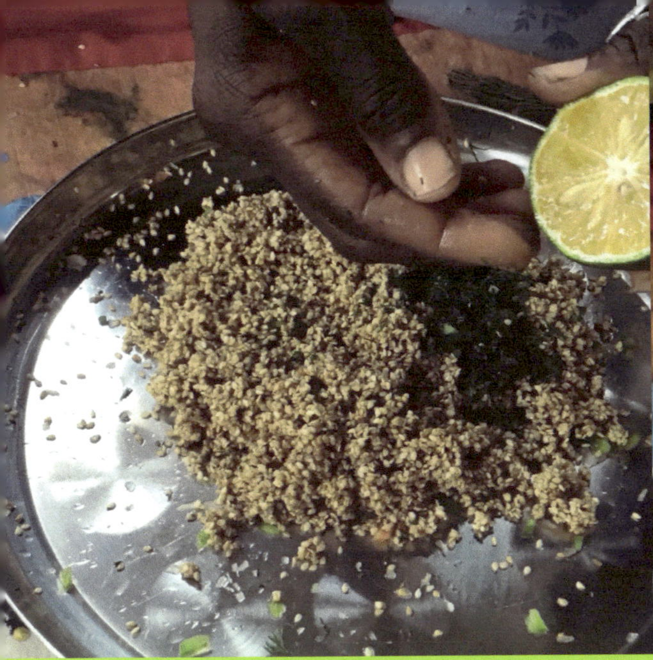

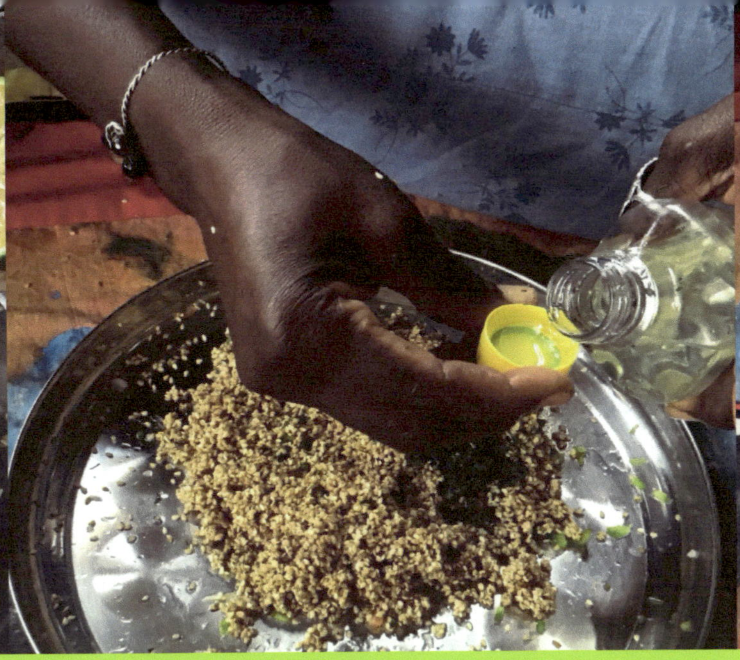

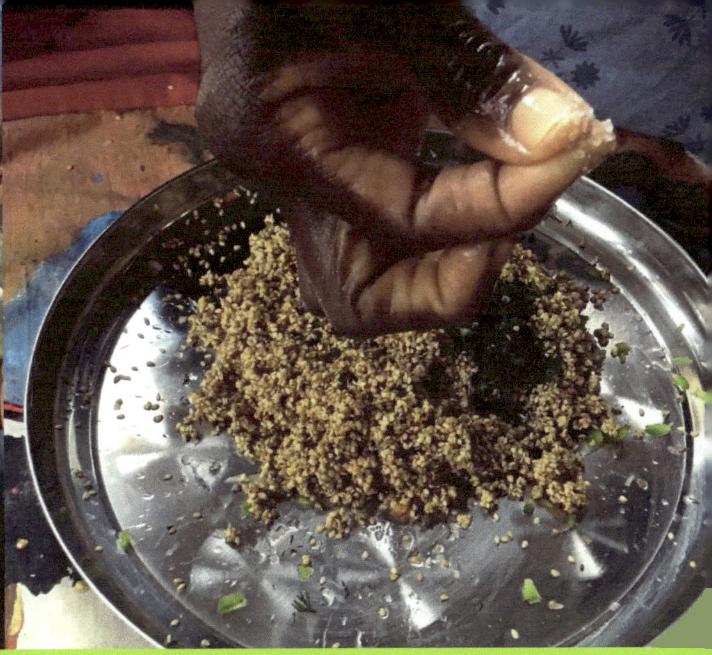

The three finalizing steps: lime to activate, oil to seal and sun-evaporated sea water to enhance.

6. Add one teaspoon fresh-squeezed lime and one teaspoon of coconut oil.

7. Add a pinch of sun-evaporated sea water.

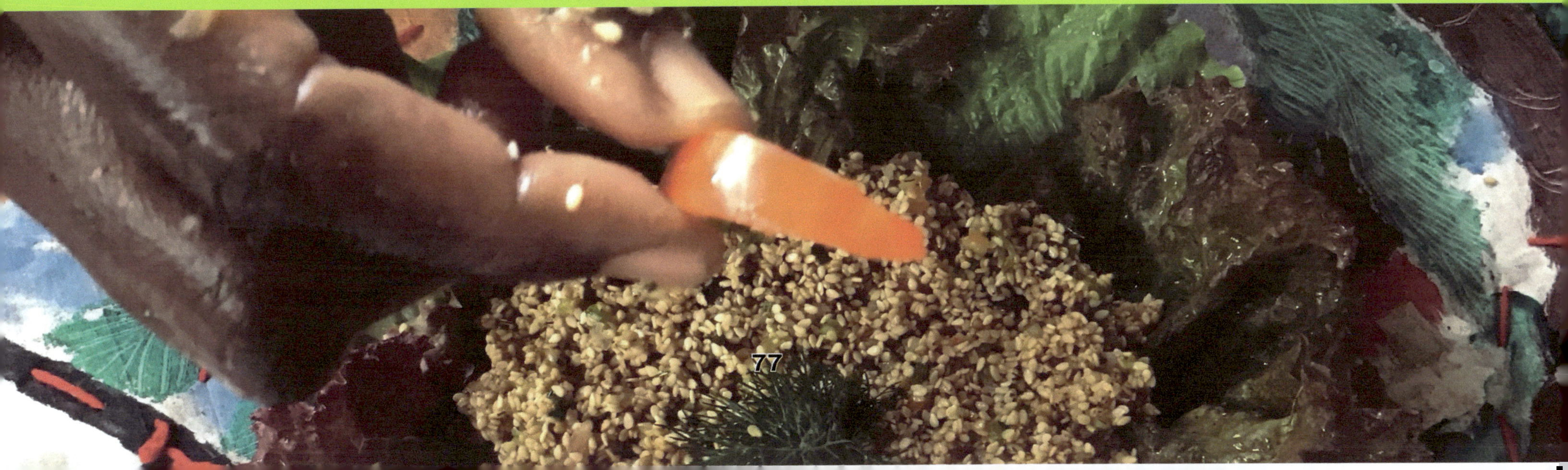

CABBAGE SAMMICH WITH BRAZIL NUT LOAF

Ingredients

brazil nuts or groundnuts (peanuts)

basil

garlic

onion

small green bell pepper

small tomato

medium celery

lettuce - romaine, green leaf, red leaf, or butter leaf

lime

coconut oil

sun-evaporated sea water

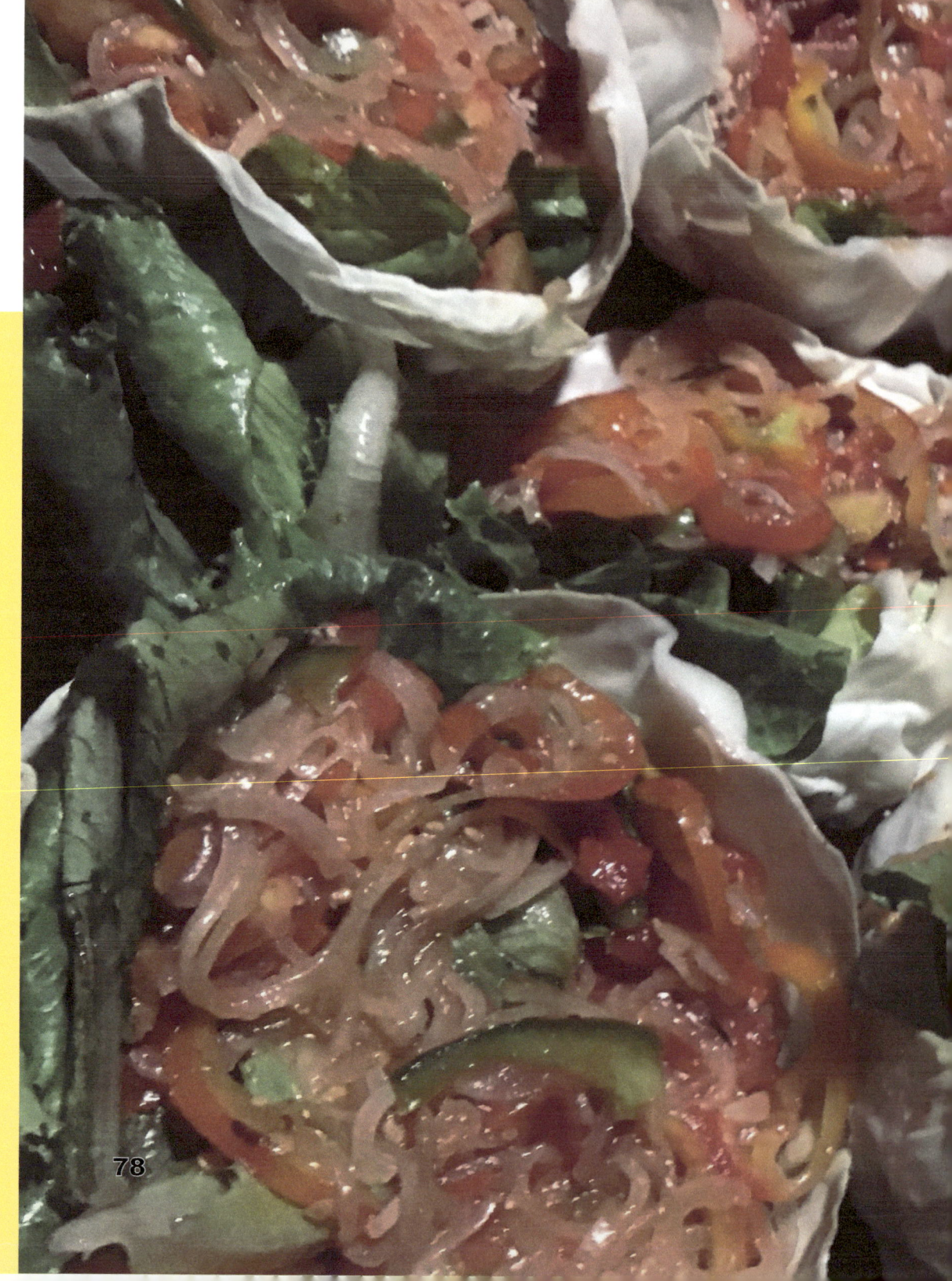

CHAPTER 7: RAW VEGAN DISHES -- GREEN IMMUNO-FUEL

Preparation Instructions

Marinated Onion topping

1. Thinly slice one half onion and one half tomato.

2. Add one teaspoon coconut oil.

3. Mix well with one teaspoon fresh-squeezed lime juice and sun-evaporated sea water.

4. Leave the onion-tomato mixture to marinate as the topping for this wonderful cabbage sammich that you are about to prepare.

Brazil-Nut-Loaf Stuffing

1. Dice one half onion, one quarter bell pepper, one half tomato, one third stalk celery. Place in a large mixing bowl and set to the side.

2. Pre-soak and rinse one handful of brazil nuts. Again, we note that it is a necessity that you follow the soaking techniques as detailed in the Green Book (*Raw and Living Foods* Book) mentioned previously.

3. Place brazil nuts in food processor. Add 3 or 4 leaves basil and one clove fresh garlic. Pulse the food processor nine times and then blend until the nut texture is grainy.

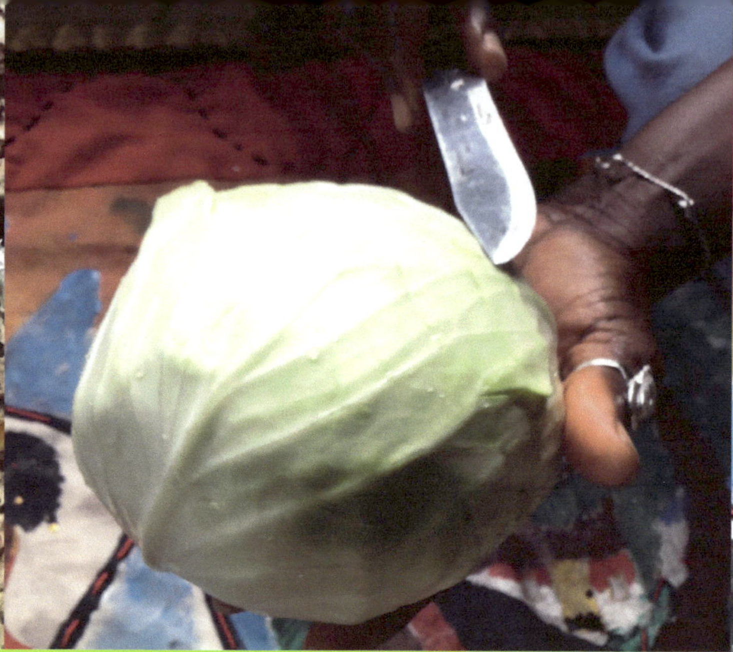

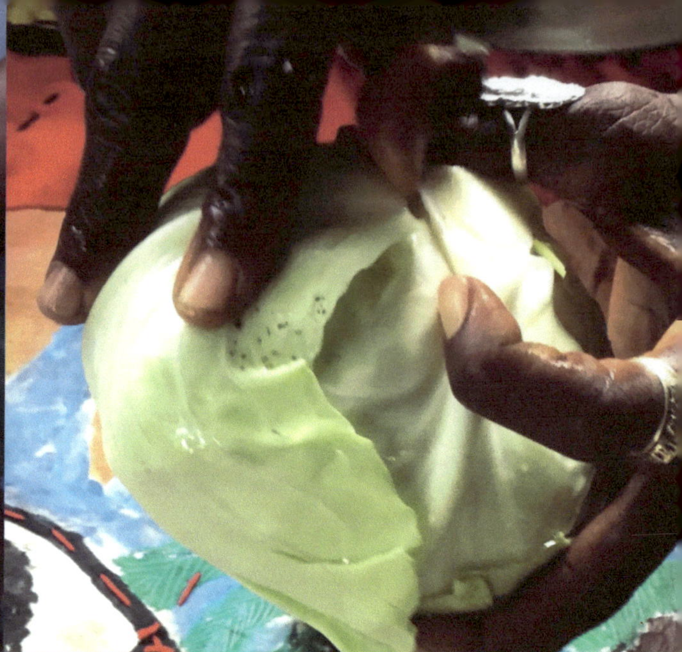

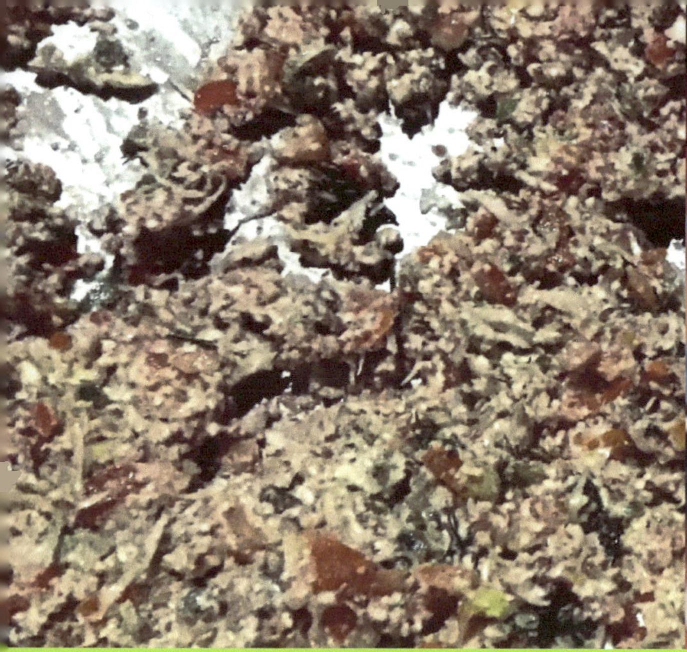

4. Add Brazil-nut mixture to diced vegetables. Add one pinch of sun-evaporated sea water. Mix very well.

5. Gently remove one whole cabbage leaf from the head of the cabbage. Place the nut mixture inside the cabbage leaf on one side, and place one whole lettuce leaf on the other side. In Belize, there is a very delicious lettuce that we prefer above all others called "local lettuce" or "ball-head lettuce."

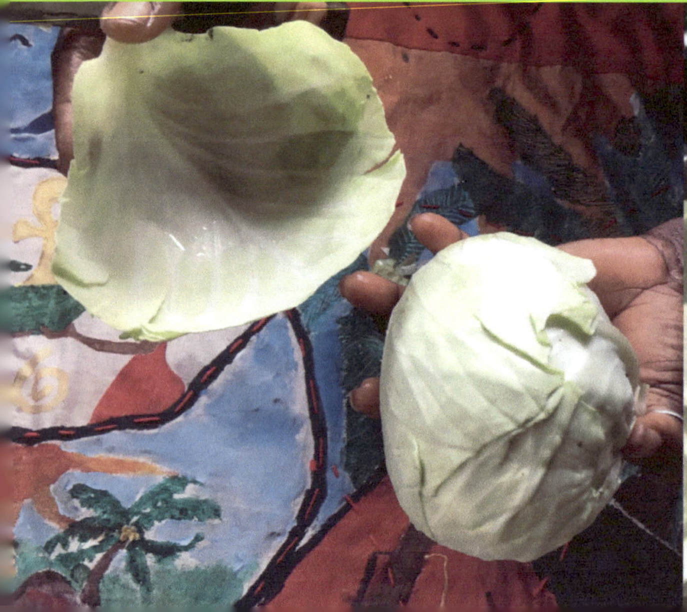

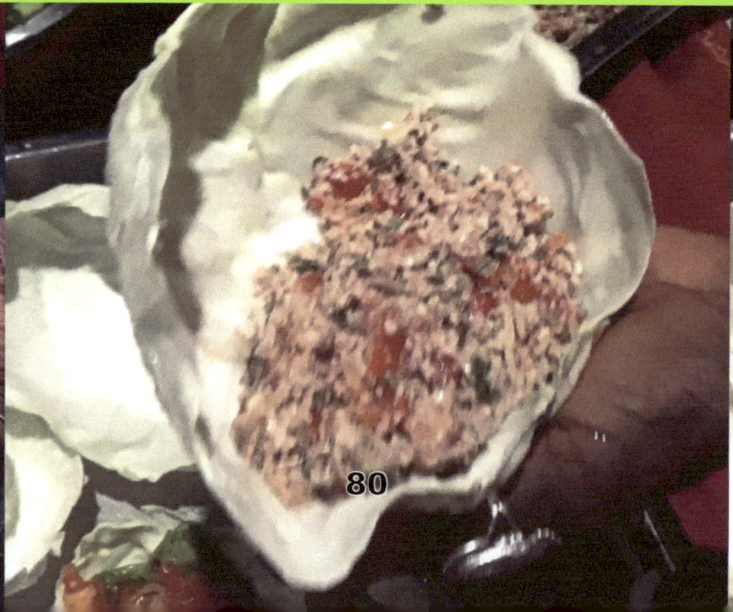

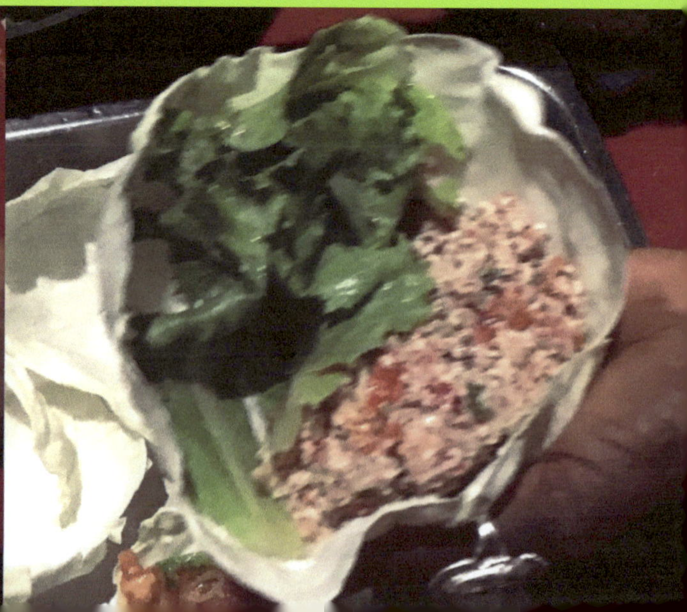

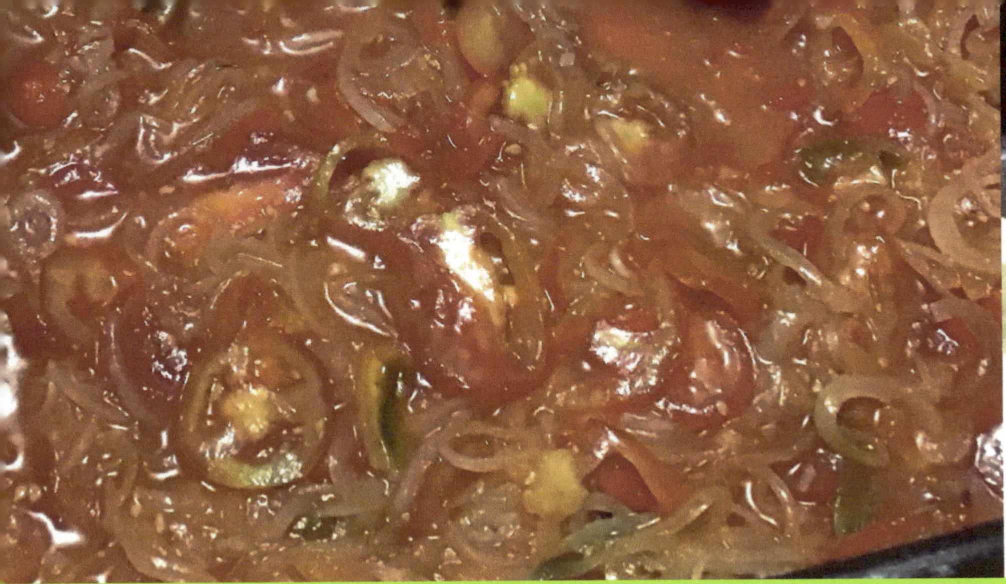

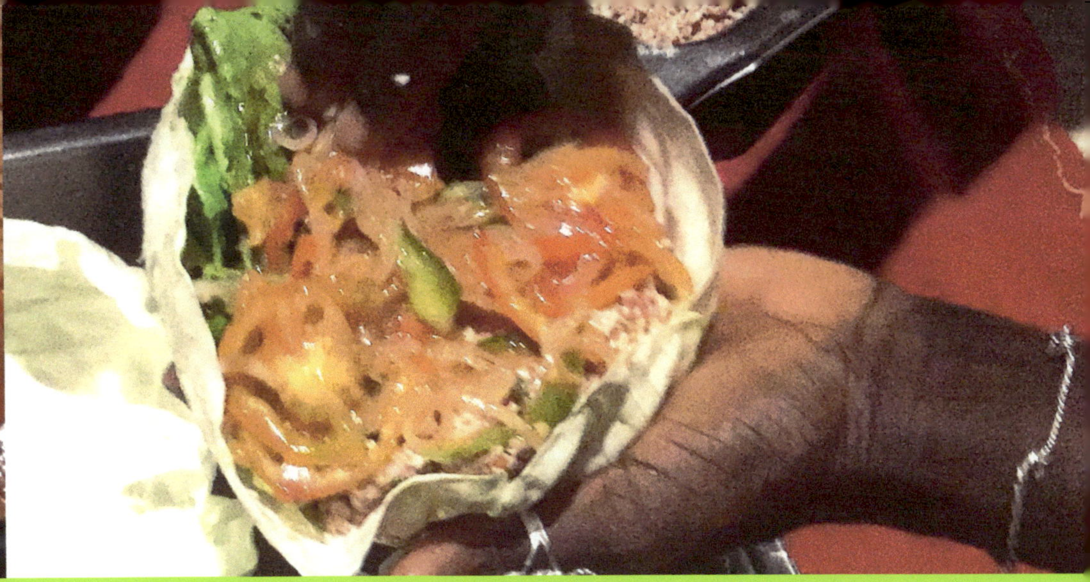

6. Spread the marinated-onion topping over the cabbage sammich. Prepare for the most delicious bite of wholesome raw and living energy that one can imagine.

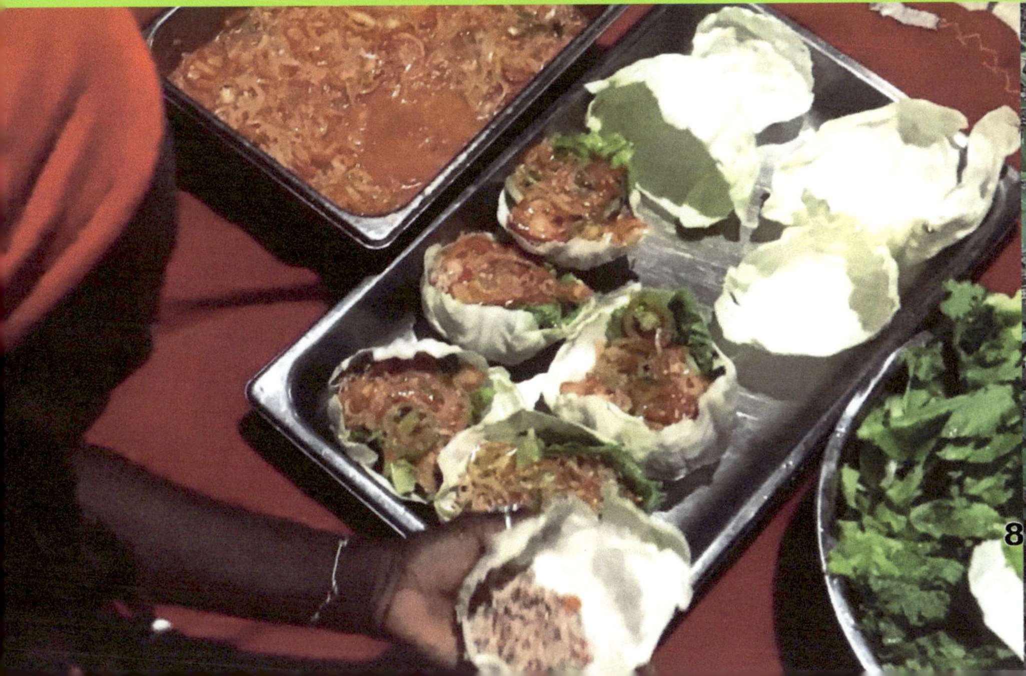

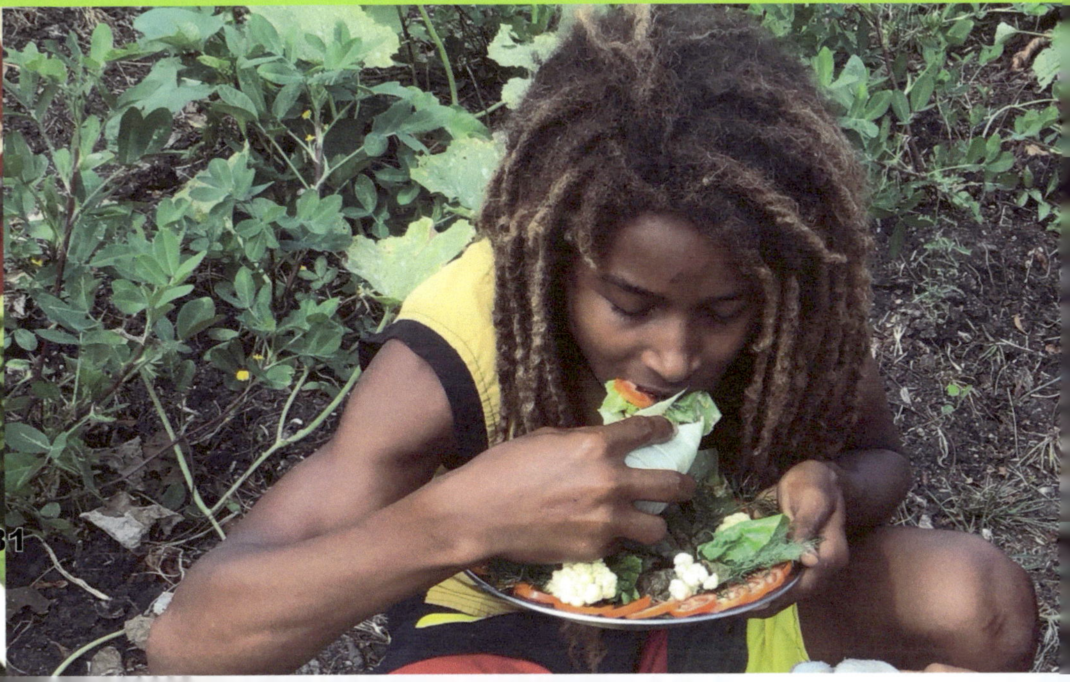

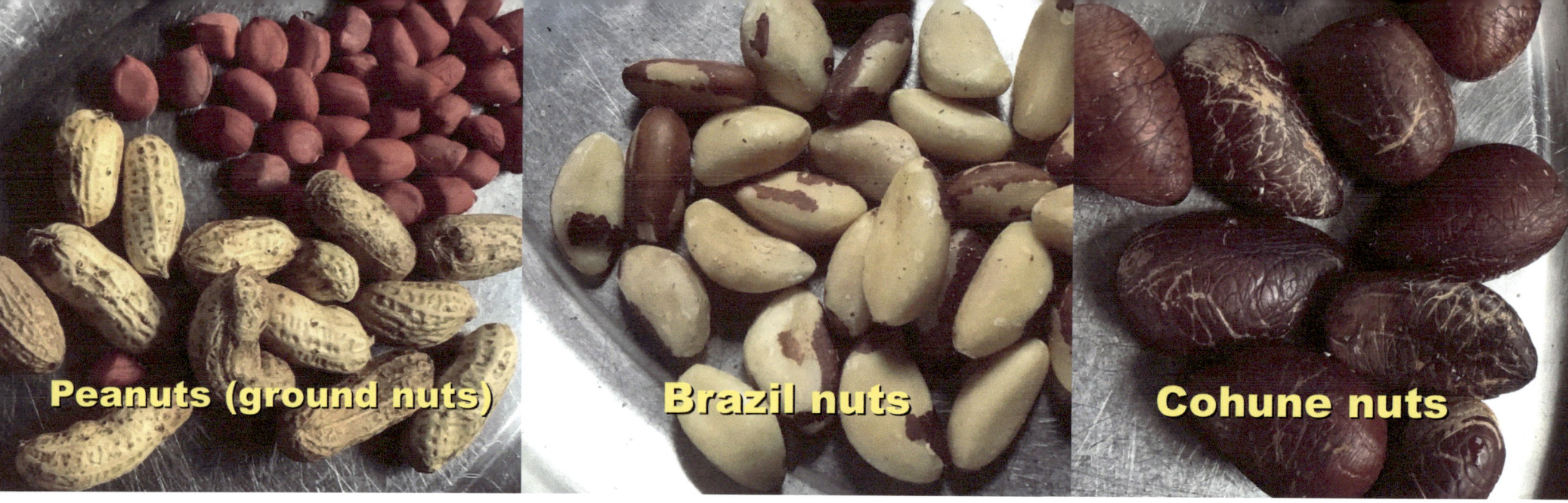

Research studies have shown that deficiency of high-quality protein can result in depletion of immune cells, inability of the body to make antibodies, and other immune-related problems.

Featured Ingredient: Brazil nuts

Brazil nuts are high in calcium, iron, phosphorus and potassium. They also contain vitamin B_1. Their calcium content makes them good for teeth and bones. As with all nuts, Brazil nuts serve as an excellent food for pregnancy, nursing mothers and for children and growing adults and are good generally for relieving nutritional deficiencies.

Peanuts (ground nuts)

Peanuts or ground nuts, as they are identified among the Kwatamani First Genesis Tribe, are reported to have more protein than any nut, containing more than 30 essential vitamins and minerals, and are a good source of fiber and beneficial fats. They are high in vitamins B_3 and B_5, inositol and magnesium. Peanuts also contain significant amounts of vitamins B_1, B_2 and E, calcium, iron and potassium.

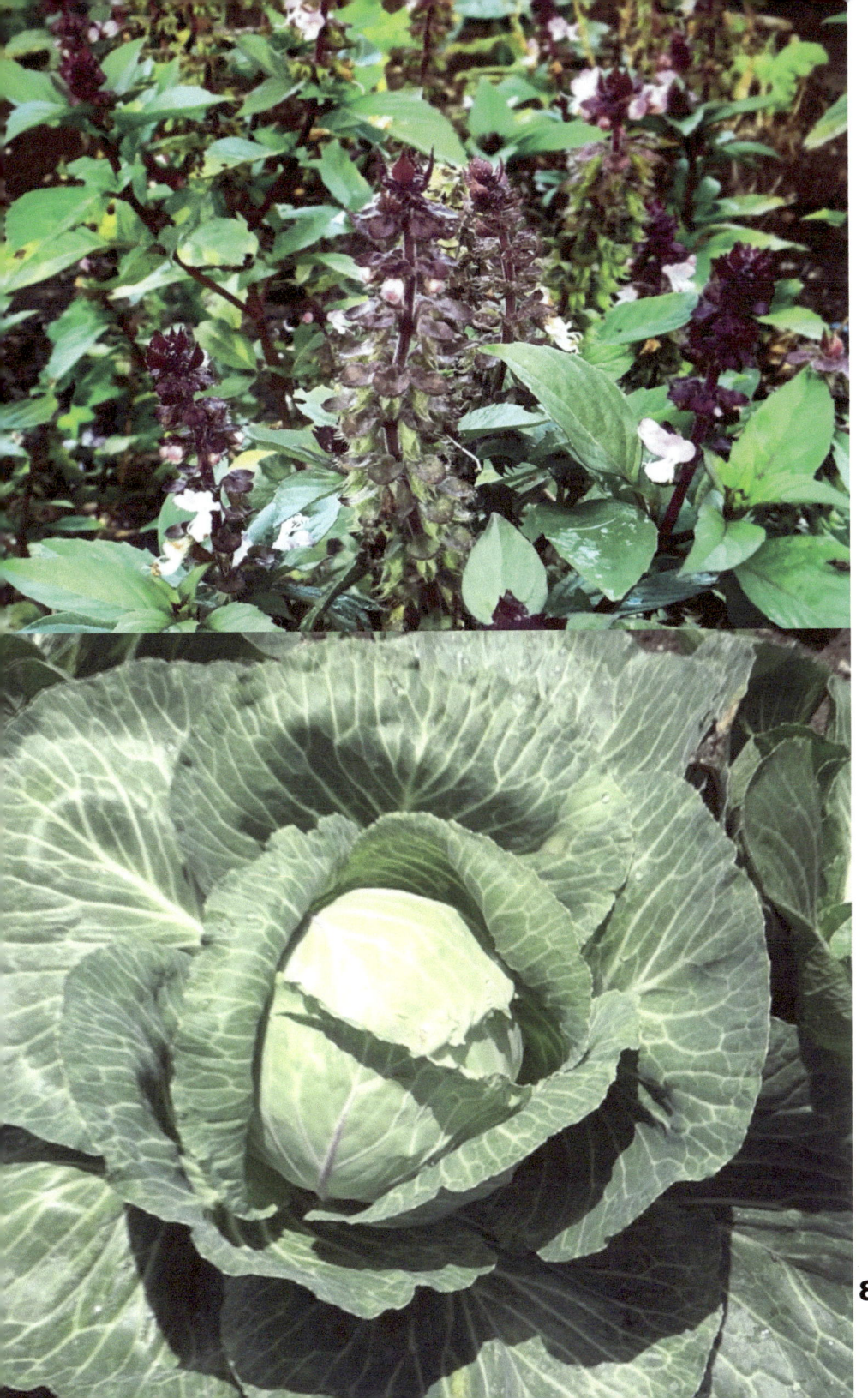

Featured Ingredient: Basil

Basil is good for indigestion, fevers, colds, flu, kidney and bladder troubles, headaches, cramps, nausea, vomiting, constipation and nervous conditions. It is used for relieving gas, reducing fever, as a blood purifier, stimulant and diuretic and for calming the nerves.

Featured Ingredient: Cabbage

Cabbage is high in vitamins B_5, B_6, C, K, chlorine, iodine, silicon, sulfur and potassium. It also contains selenium and vitamin E. Cabbage is an excellent cleanser, particularly for the mucous membranes of the stomach and intestines. It is also a good blood cleanser and aids in maintaining healthy teeth, gums, hair, nails and bones.

Cabbage is also helpful treating kidney and bladder disorders. My recommendation that cabbage juice be used for treating ulcers has been proven very successful over the years, especially when combined with a whole, live diet.

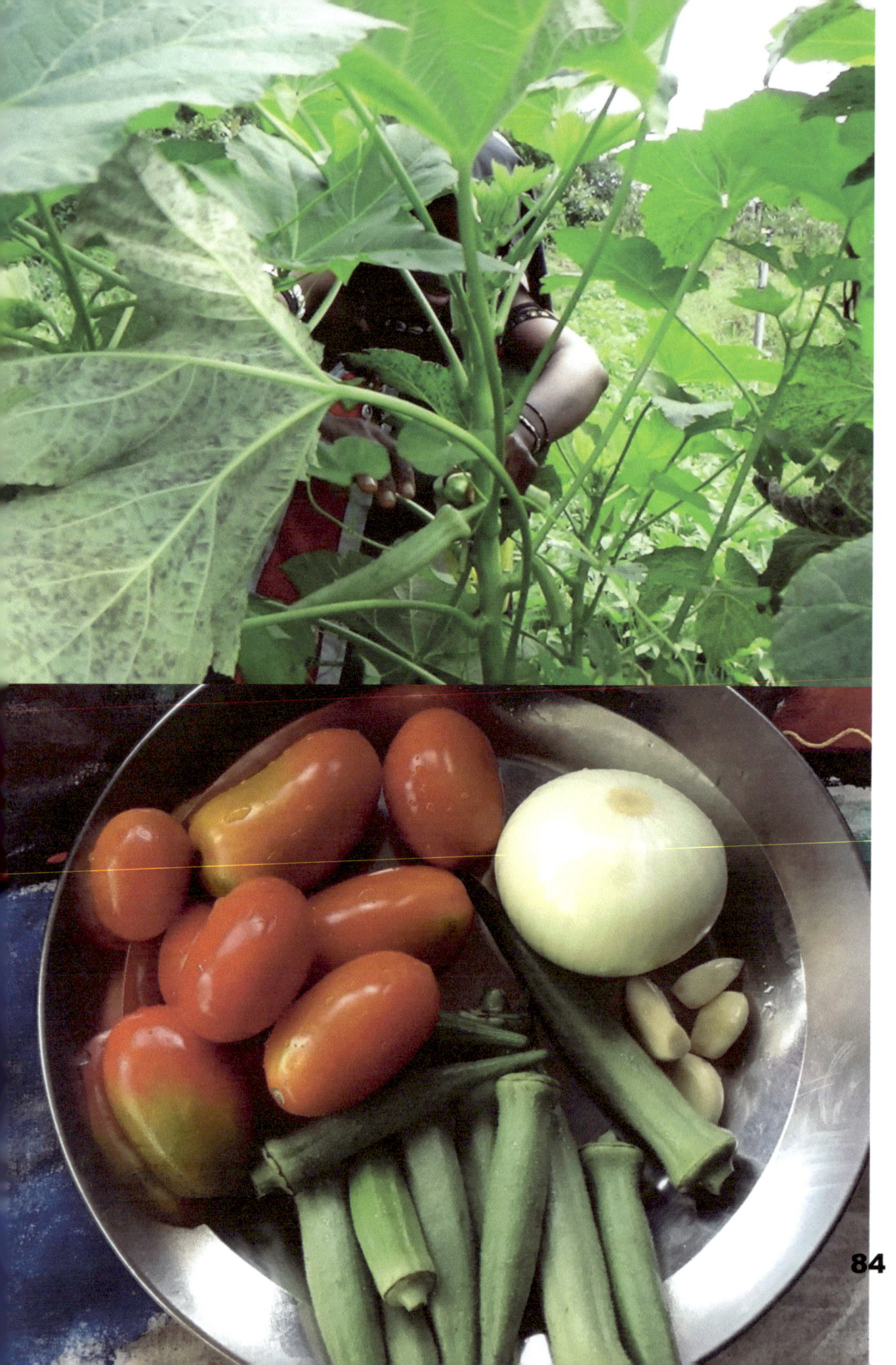

If you have been one to say, "Ugh, I don't like okra," we have a tasty dish that just might change your mind.

OKRA IN THE RAW

Ingredients

okra – 3 to 4 whole okra, depending on your appetite

tomato, medium

onion, medium

garlic

lime

coconut oil

sun-evaporated sea water

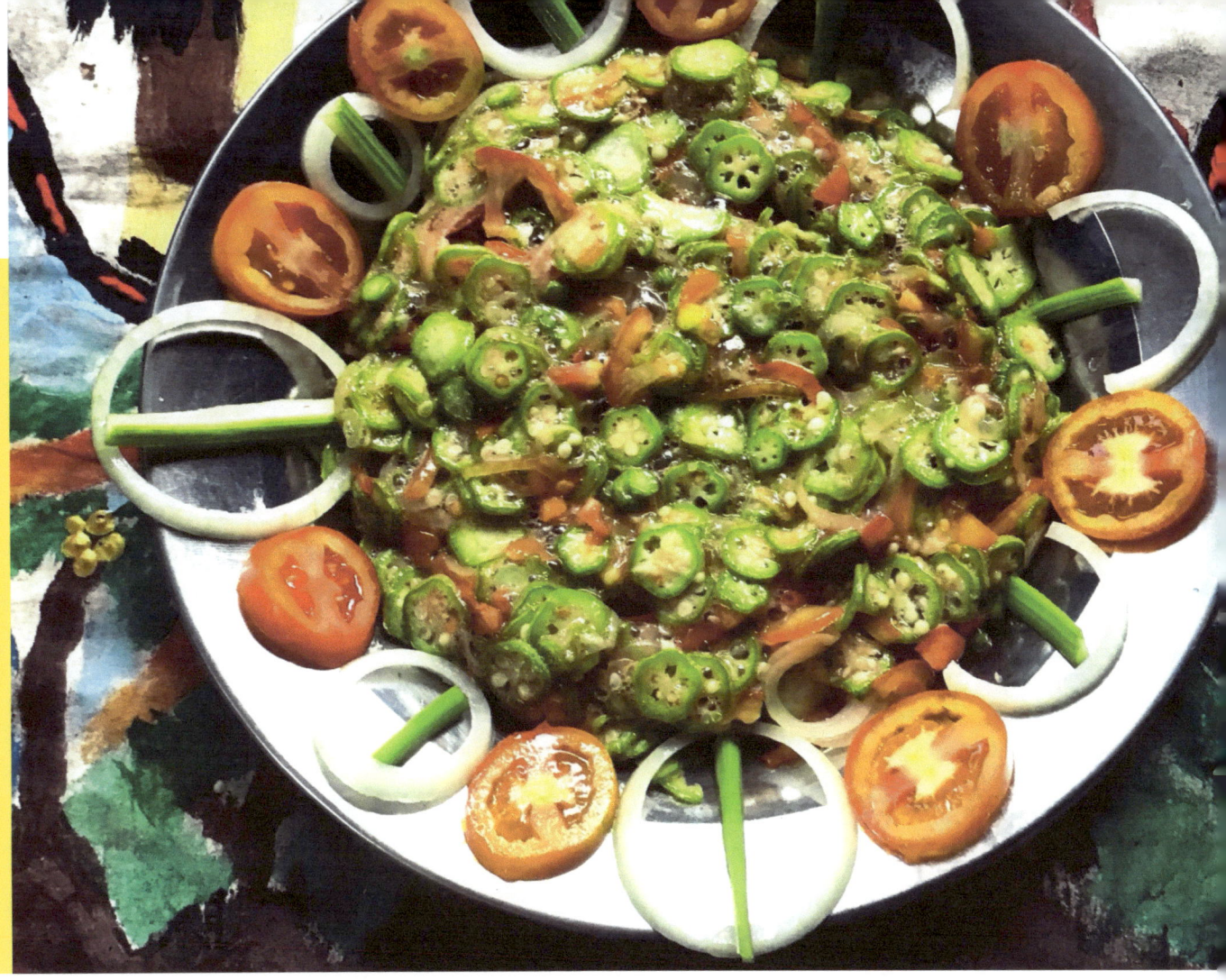

"We remind you that the ancestral wisdom among the Akan states that Man, He and She, is a spirit or energy presence made of three elements. The first element is the Okra which refers to the innermost being, the essence of the person. Unfortunately, one can only tap into the ancestral soul of okra by consuming it whole and natural, raw and living. Now, ain't that something". KRIST Text, p. 234

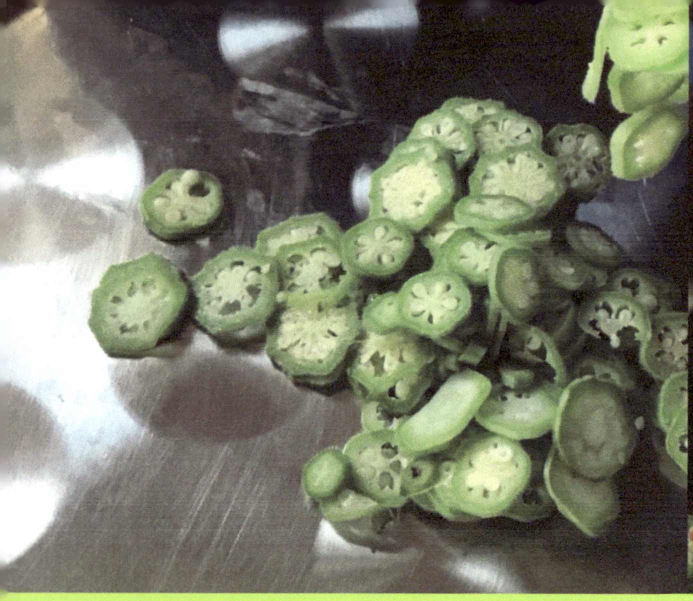

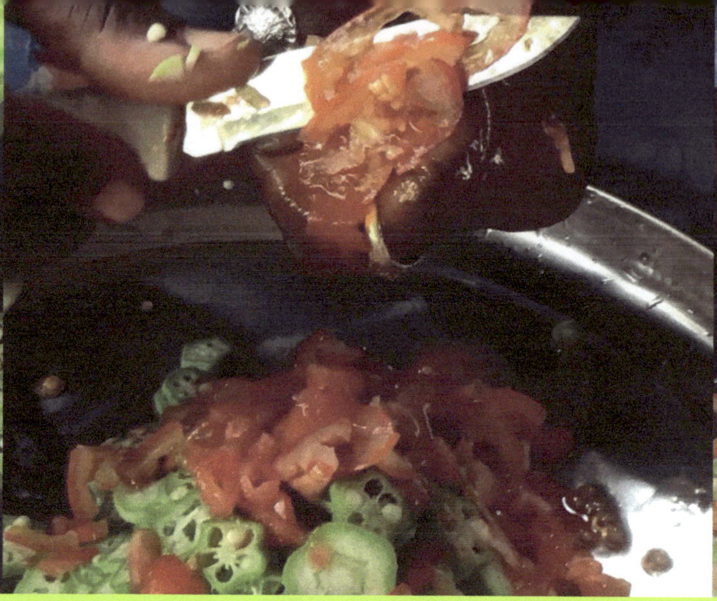

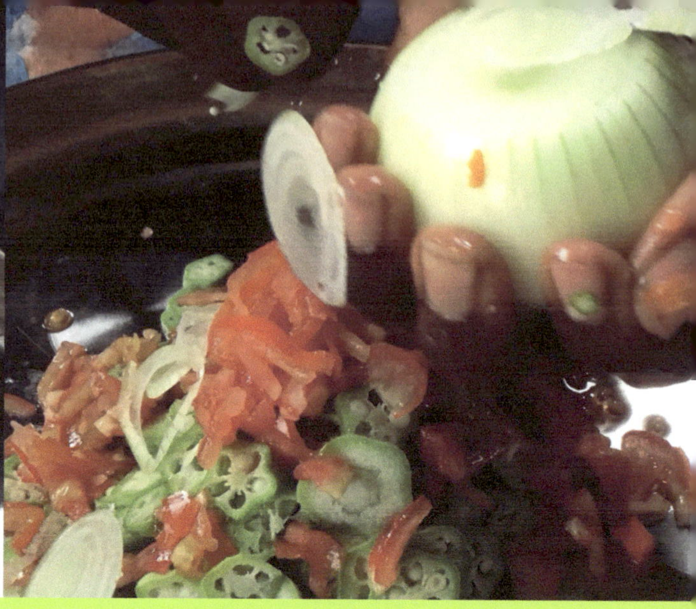

1. Slice the okra as thin as the cover of this book, if you can, and place the slices in a mixing bowl.

2. Finely slice half of a medium-sized tomato and one quarter of the onion. Add to okra.

3. Use a fine grater or press one clove of a medium-sized garlic and add to the mix. If you are not a strong garlic-lover like we are, then you may want to use a little less garlic.

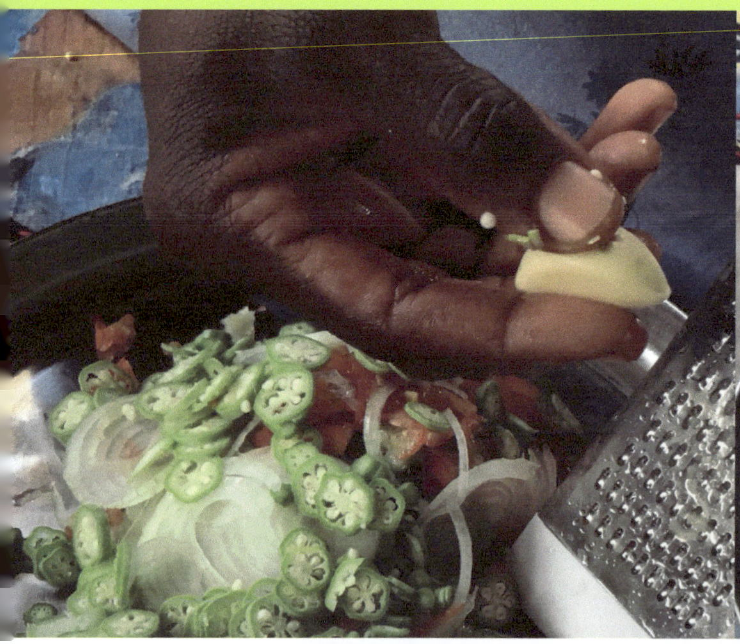

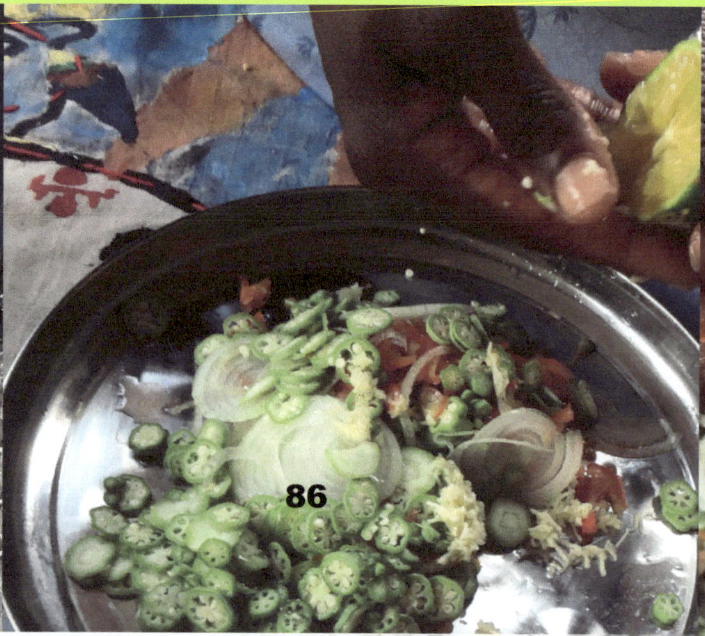

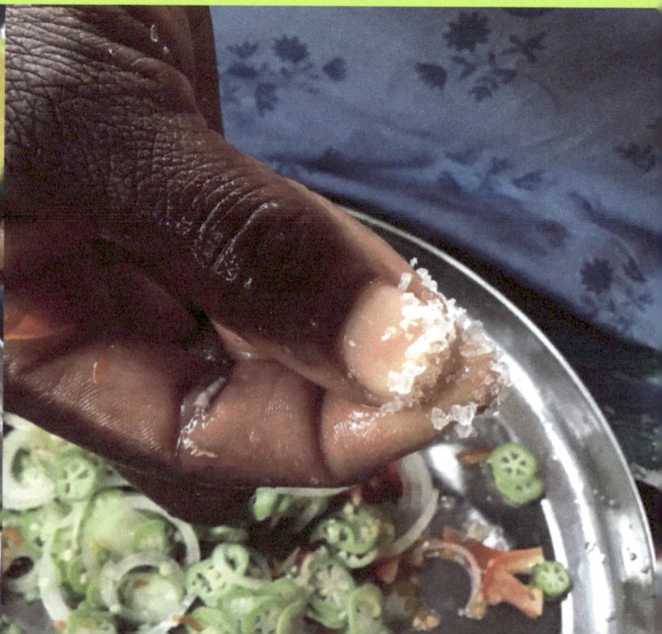

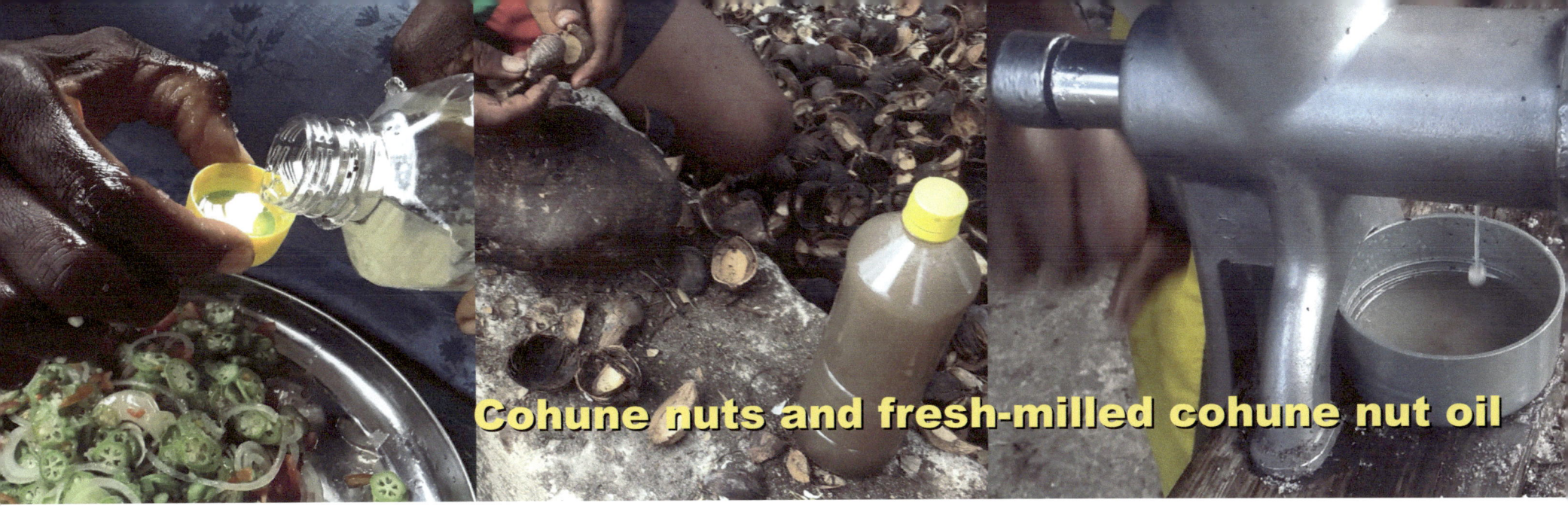

Cohune nuts and fresh-milled cohune nut oil

4. Add one and a half teaspoons of coconut oil.

Please make sure your oil is as raw and fresh as possible, preferably home-made. Any cooked or otherwise unnaturally prepared oil – using anything other than a first-cold-pressed process – will deteriorate essential nutrient factors of the oil.

Please, do not put trauma on your ingestive system, and do not traumatize the living matter of your food. You will be forever grateful to Mother Earth and the supreme energies of wind, rain, and sun. At all points in time, remember that you are preparing food for thought, literally and figuratively.

We are able to enjoy the cohune palm trees growing in our Garden Sanctuary and harvest the cohune nuts. Extracting the cohune nut from its shell takes a bit of work, but our youth have devised a simple rock method that works well. We then use a hand mill to squeeze the fresh cohune nut oil.

CODE GREEN: HIDDEN POWERS OF THE GARDEN TARGETING THE IMMUNE SYSTEM

5. Add one and a half teaspoons of fresh-squeezed lime juice (the natural body antiseptic) and a pinch of sun-evaporated sea water.

6. Mix gently until the okra juices are well-blended. This dish is pretty simple. The same basic steps can be applied to many other vegetables, such as zucchini or eggplant. Experiment and you will get some tasty results. Again, measure your stomach and mix your vegetables according to your flavor-tasting desires for that day. Find a nice comfortable seat to meditate as you eat this life-infusing treat.

Featured Ingredient: Okra

Okra is high in calcium, sodium and potassium and contains vitamins A, B_3 (niacin) and C and small traces of B_1, B_2, iron, sulfur and phosphorus. Okra is good for treating stomach ulcers and inflammation of the lungs (pleurisy) and the colon (colitis). Okra has been recommended in cases of sore throat and obesity.

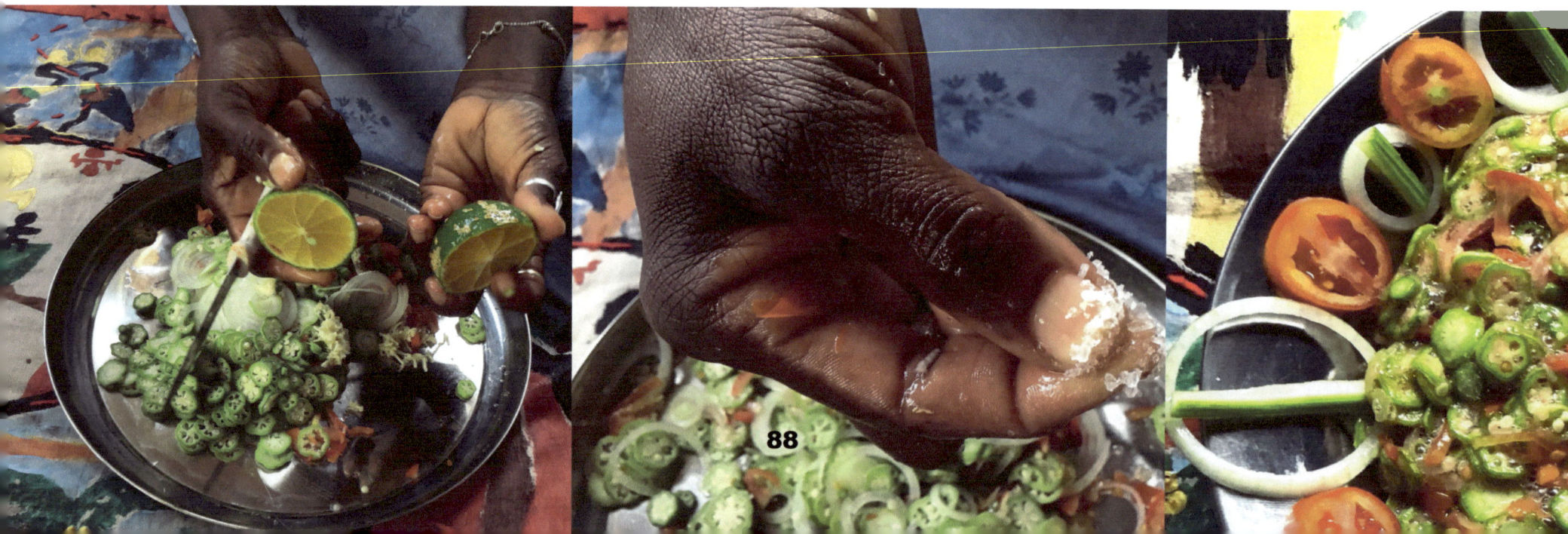

CHIA FRUIT PUDDING

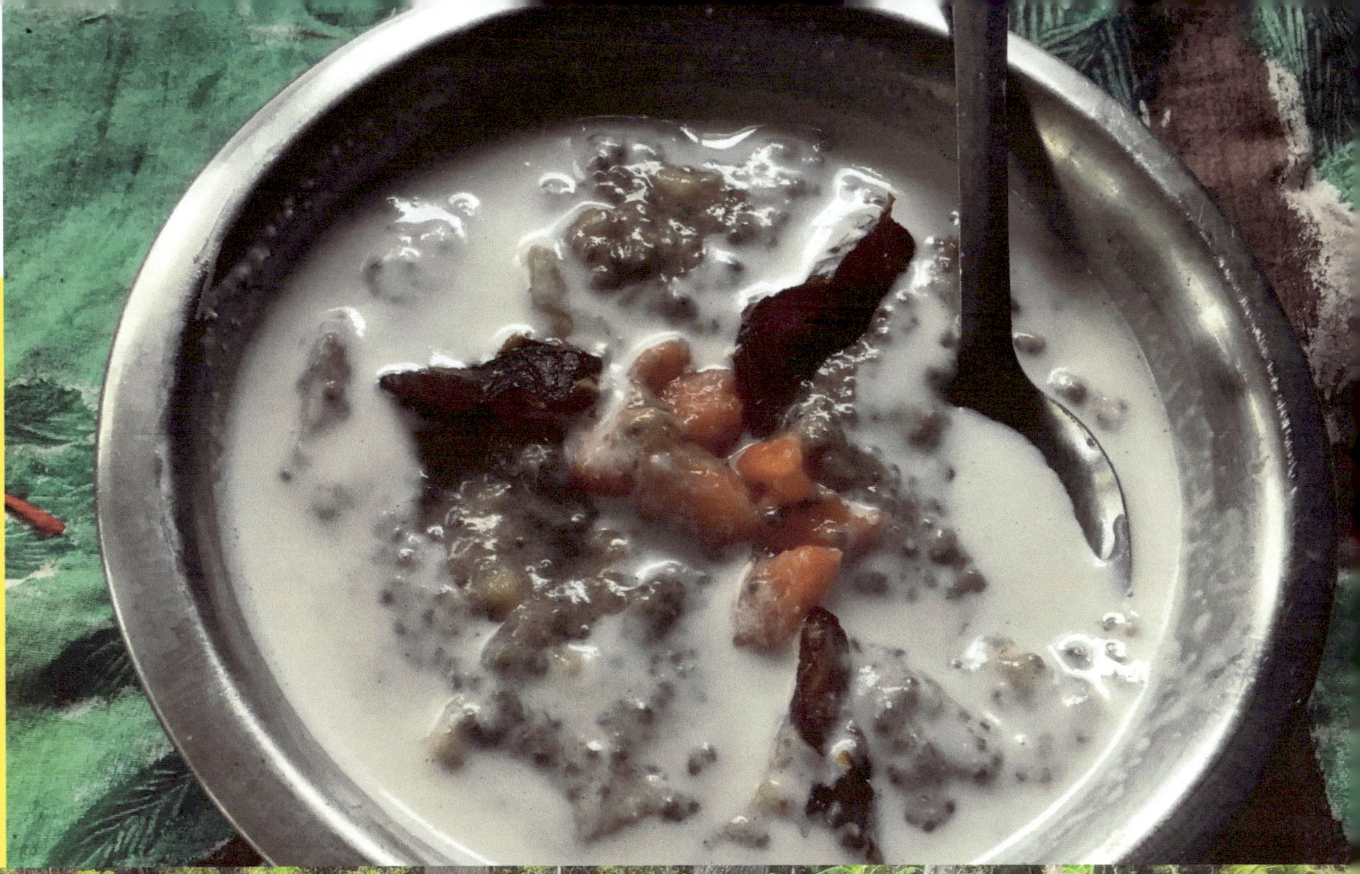

Ingredients

chia seeds

coconut

bananas

pineapple

papaya

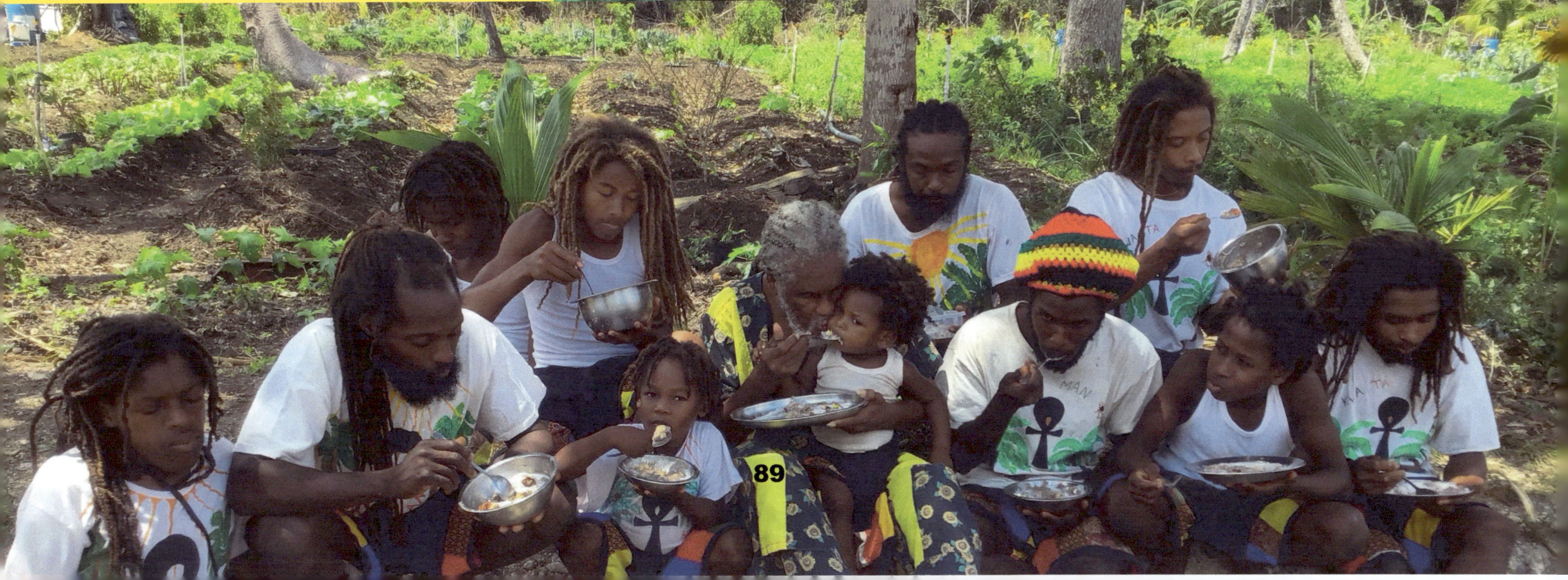

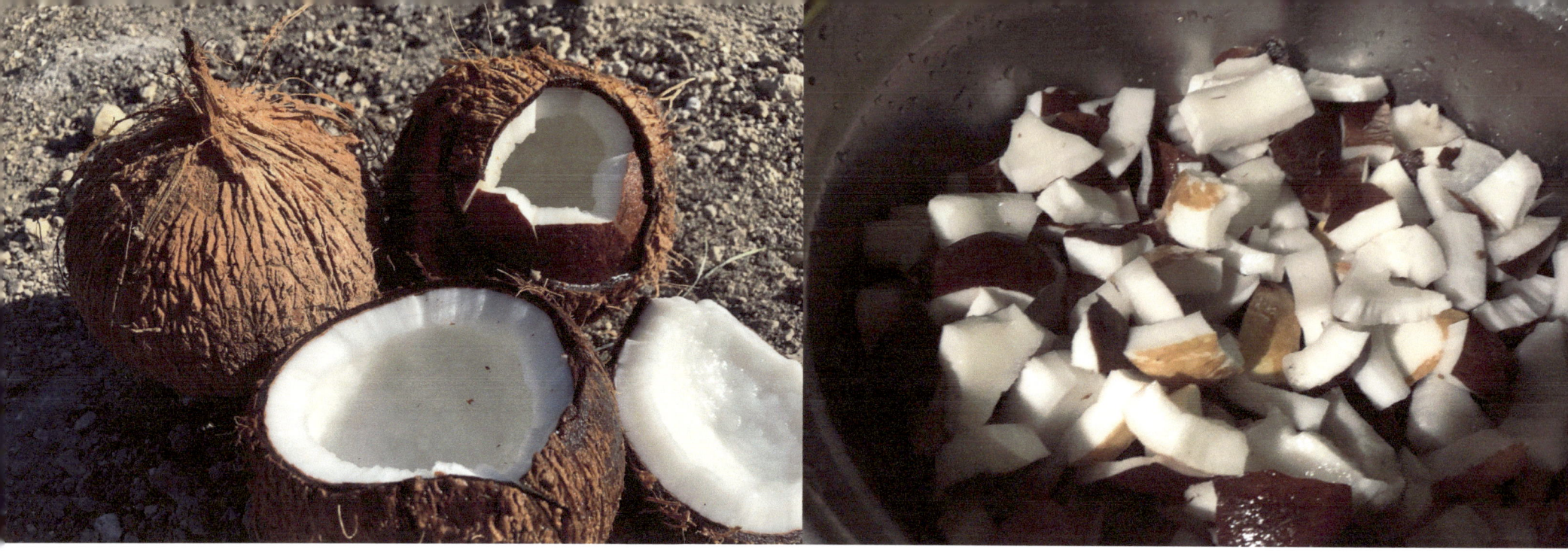

1. Crack a hard, dry coconut and pour off the coconut water. Scoop out the coconut meat from the hard outer shell. Chop the coconut meat into small pieces and rinse them well with spring water. Put the chopped coconut pieces in a big bowl.

2. Juice the coconut pieces with a juicer to extract the thick coconut milk/cream. You will not need the coconut chaff that remains for this dish. Save a portion of the coconut milk for after the chia fruit pudding is done.

3. Place the remaining coconut milk and banana pieces into a blender and blend until smooth, making what we call banana cream sauce that will be used to mix with the tropical fruit selection.

4. For this recipe, we use bananas or ripe plantain. Dice the bananas, pineapple and papaya in a bowl. Pour the dry chia seeds on top of the diced fruit.

CHAPTER 7: RAW VEGAN DISHES -- GREEN IMMUNO-FUEL

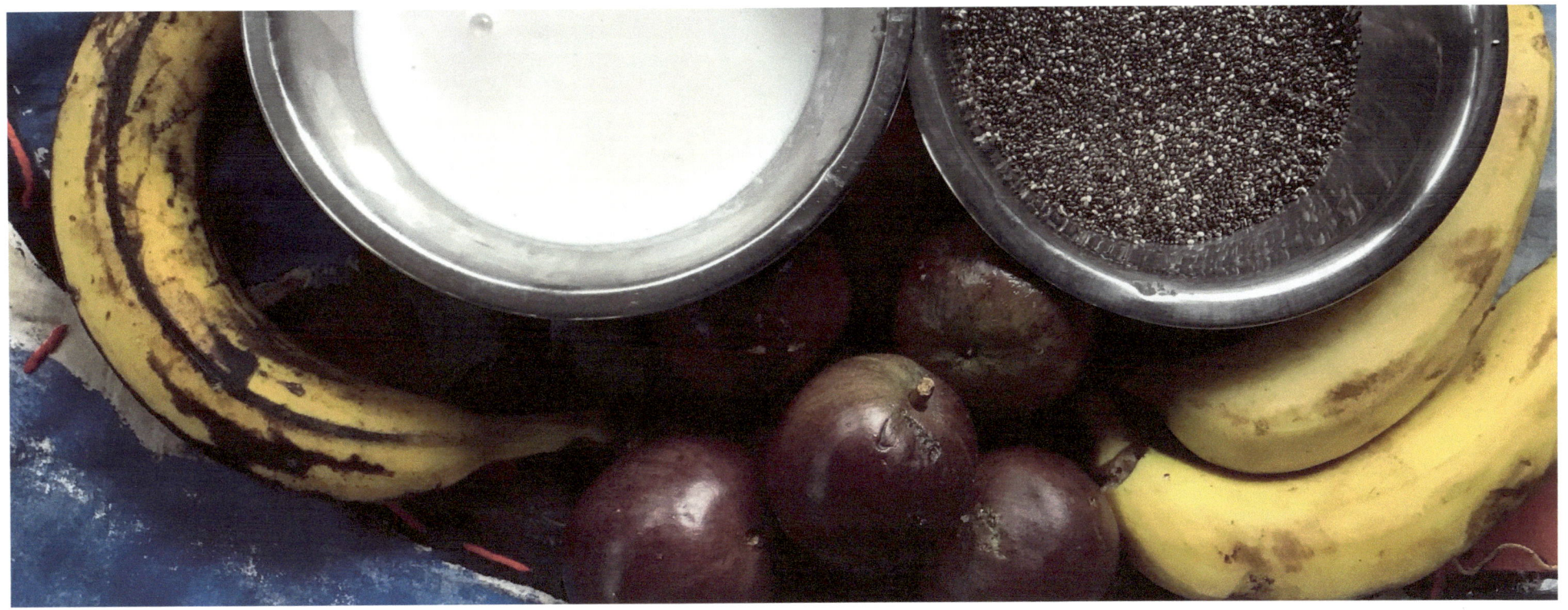

5. Pour the banana cream sauce over the chia seeds and diced fruit. Mix well.

You will need to wait just a few minutes for the chia fruit pudding to thicken. You can now pour the coconut milk over the top and add extra diced fruit as a topping.

Featured Ingredient: Chia Seeds

Chia seeds are known to be packed full of antioxidants, proteins, Omega-3 fatty acids, vitamins, and minerals such as calcium, zinc and iron.

CODE GREEN: HIDDEN POWERS OF THE GARDEN TARGETING THE IMMUNE SYSTEM

Featured Ingredient: Banana

Bananas are best noted for being high in potassium. They also contain substantial amounts of vitamin A, the B vitamins, especially B_6, biotin, calcium, magnesium, manganese, phosphorus, sulfur, chlorine and sodium. After reviewing the vitamin and mineral content of bananas, I'm sure you can see why I identify bananas as a super food. If you could have the experience of having a banana plantation and witnessing their process from birth to maturity, you would definitely walk away with a new consciousness about food birth, and you would definitely want to eat more bananas.

Bananas have a soothing effect on the digestive system and are very calming to the central nervous system. They are also an excellent energy food…. It should be well noted that bananas are one of those foods that serve womanhood well, while also being of tremendous assistance in increasing the energy level of the man. Bananas are best eaten when they are spotted. This is when they are the sweetest. When they go past that stage, they can serve in the same capacity to sweeten as medjool or honey ball dates.

Bananas are also a staple food of the Kwatamani First Genesis Tribe and should be considered as a staple food of any live foodist who has the ability to access this magnificent fruit.

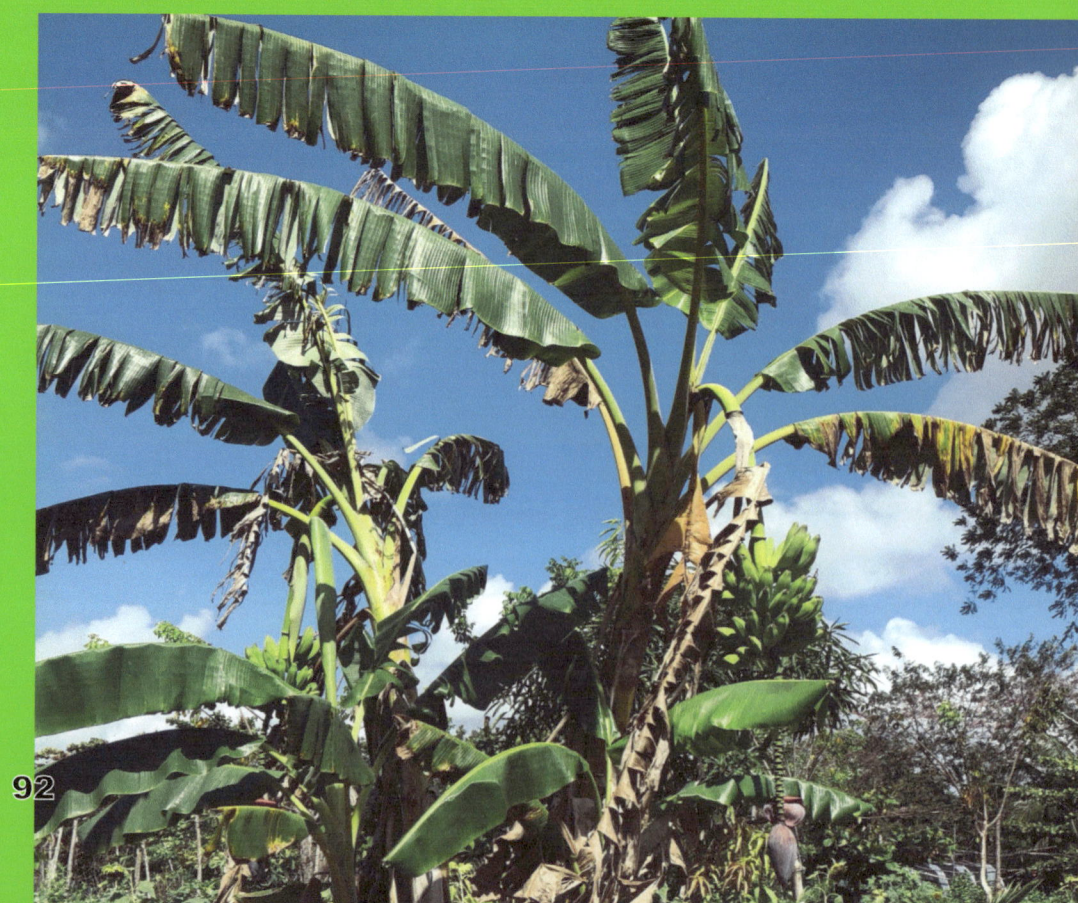

KEMETIC KUSH SUPREME: KWA-TOULI #9

Ingredients

sundried peas/legumes of choice

onion, small

green bell pepper

small tomato

lime

coconut

sun-evaporated sea water

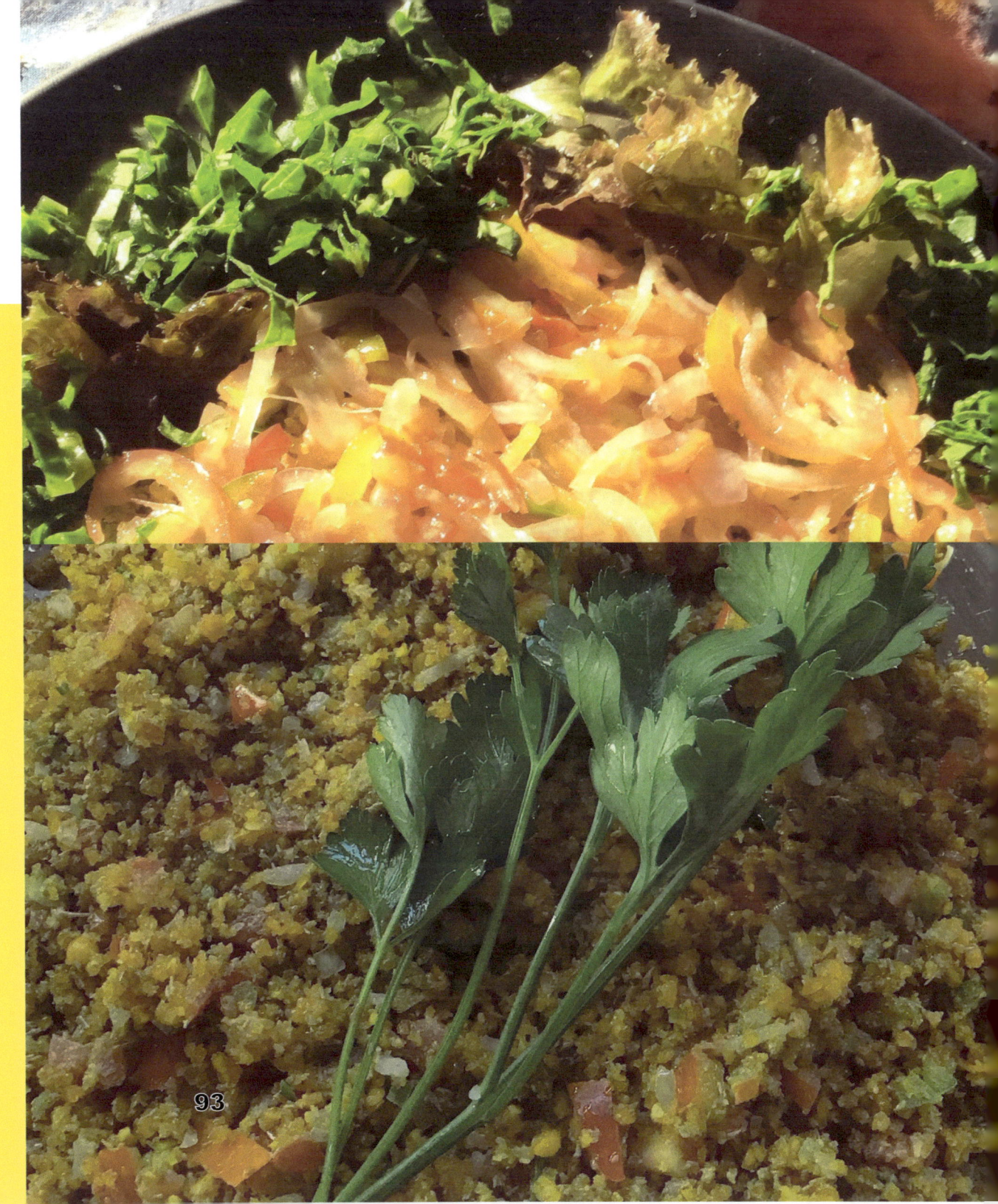

CODE GREEN: HIDDEN POWERS OF THE GARDEN TARGETING THE IMMUNE SYSTEM

This dish is popularly identified as the Kemetic Kush Supreme. It can be made using sundried peas. Lentils are a popular base. However, other dried legumes and peas will work well. There are many types: adzuki beans, black beans, black-eyed peas, broad beans (fava beans), calico beans, garbanzo beans (also called chickpeas), mung beans, navy beans, ground nuts (also called peanuts), soybeans, and others.

This dish has been with the I in I for approximately 40 years. Although we have used many different peas, beans and grains, its global popularity has continued to be rated as one of our most popular dishes.

Whether you purchase your peas or grow them, make sure that you lay them out to sun-dry well. Several hours of direct sunlight is preferred.

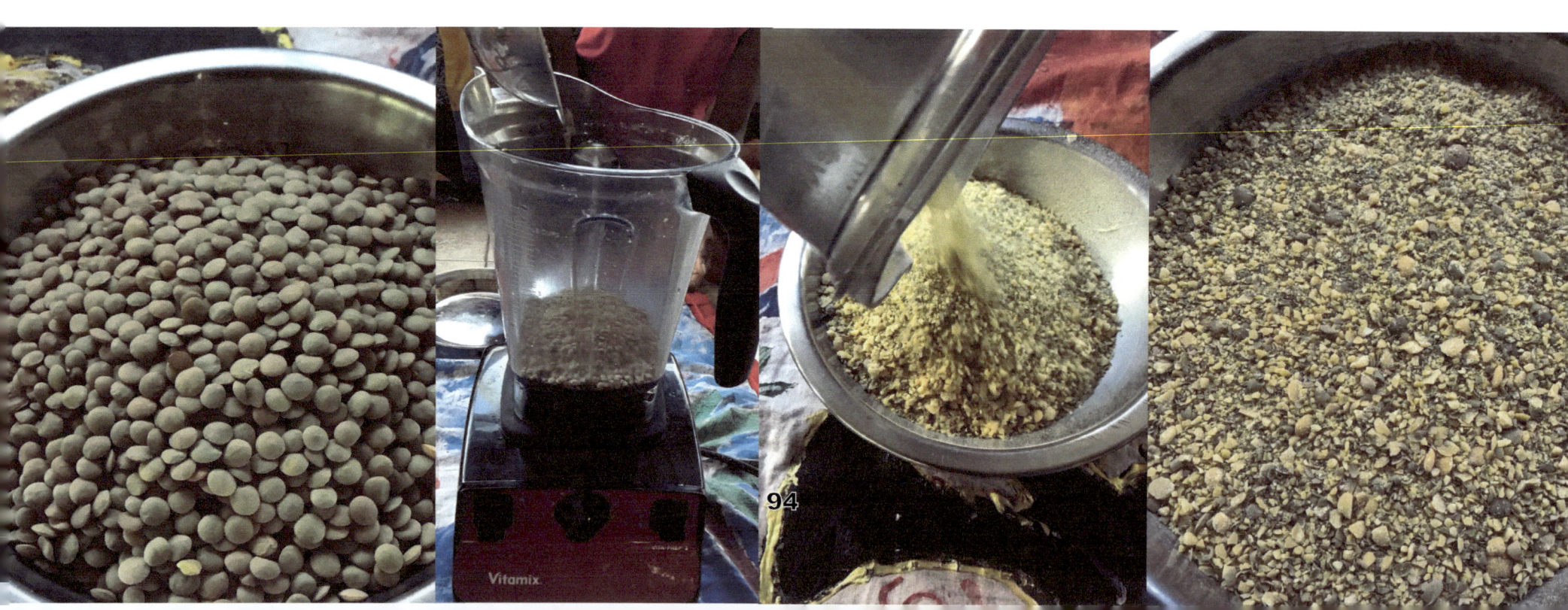

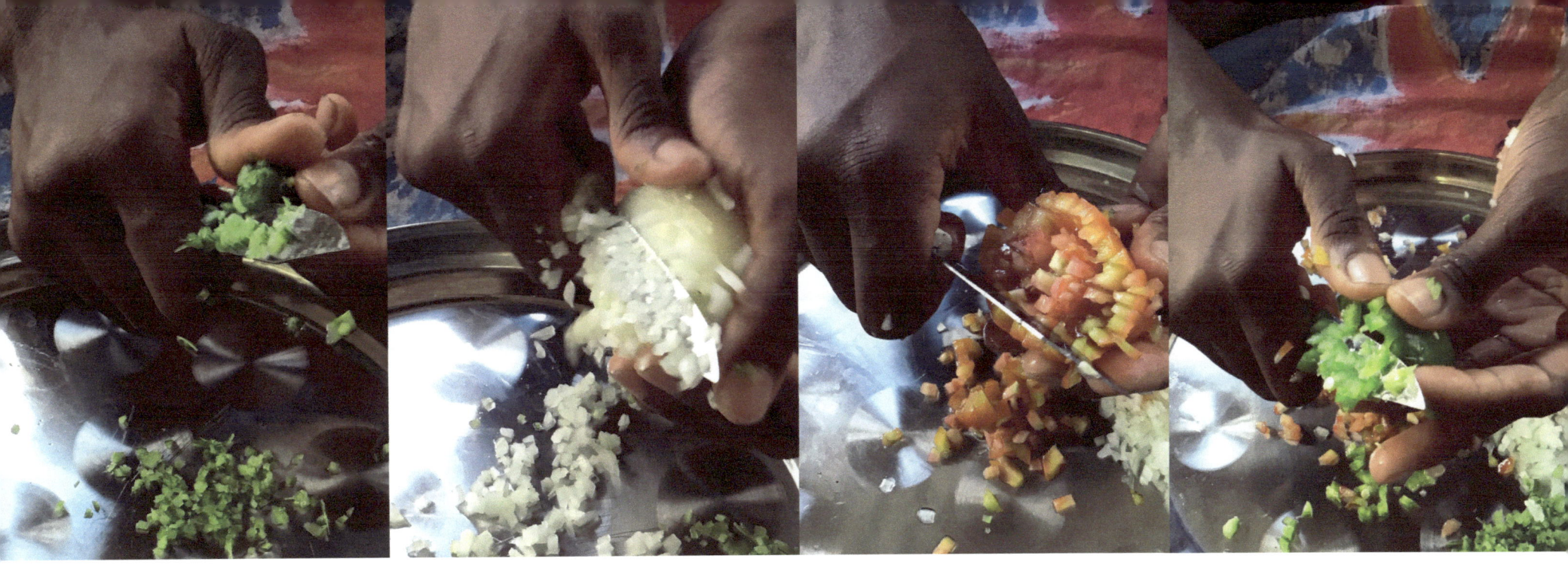

1. Put the dried peas/legumes in a blender and grind to a coarse texture.

2. Place the kush (ground peas/legumes) in a bowl and put in a little bit of spring water to soak.

3. Dice tomato, celery, bell pepper, and onion.

4. Put vegetables on top of the soaked kush.

5. Add one teaspoon lime juice, one and a half teaspoons coconut oil, and a pinch or two of sun-dried evaporated sea water. Mix well.

6. In a separate bowl, slice onions, tomato, and bell pepper. Add coconut oil, lime, and sun-dried evaporated sea water to sliced vegetables. Mix together into a marinated topping.

7. Put the kush in a bowl. Put the marinated topping over the kush. Eat and enjoy.

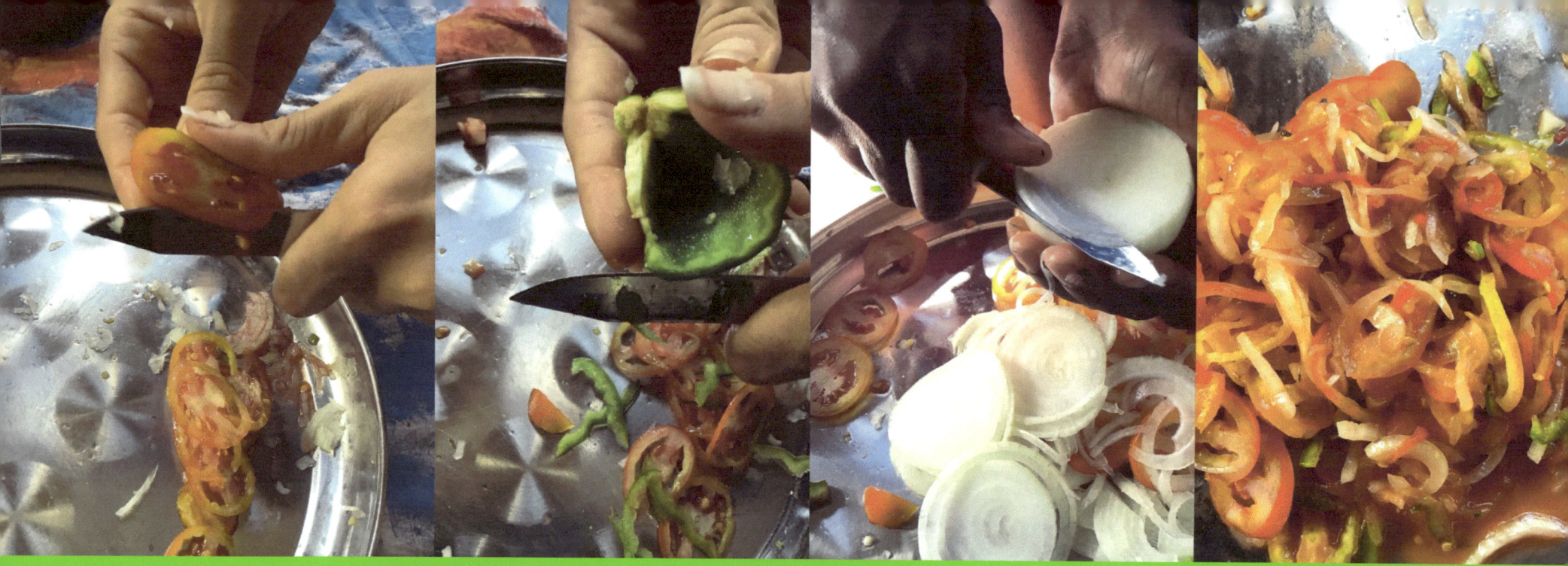

Featured Ingredient: Lentils

Lentils are noted to be a part of the legume family, providing a primary source of plant protein. The fiber content in lentils acts as a prebiotic that helps to improve intestinal health and maintains a healthy microflora environment. The soluble fiber boosts the population of good bacteria in the intestine which is linked to improved immunity, anti-inflammatory effects and even enhanced mood. This makes the body more efficient at processing waste while maximizing the nutritional content of the food ingested.

Extremely rich in immune boosting minerals, lentils provide a healthy dose of zinc, folate, copper, manganese, magnesium and selenium. Magnesium improves blood flow, oxygen and nutrients throughout the body.

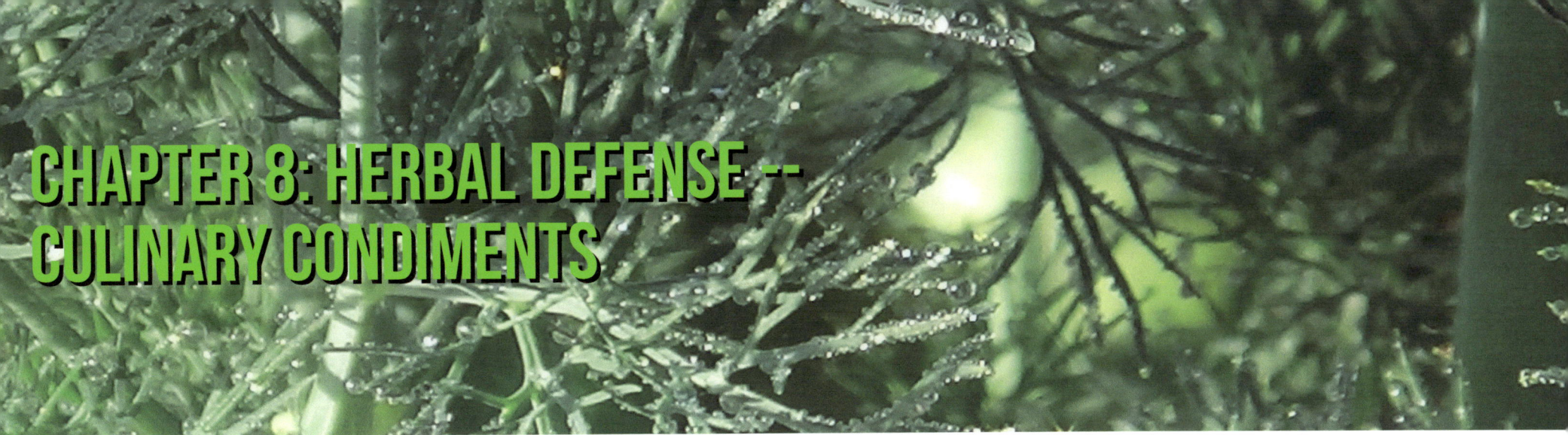

CHAPTER 8: HERBAL DEFENSE -- CULINARY CONDIMENTS

Genesis 1:29 "Behold, I have given you every herb- bearing seed, which is upon the face of the earth and every tree that has seed-yielding fruit — to you it shall be for food." As we have stated, the Kemetic Naga Priesthood traditions far pre-date the coming of those warring, flesh-consuming, sheep-herding tribes and clans who raided and invaded our sacred ancestral garden-culture lands. We note that ancient Garden-Culture River-Valley civilizations have been the carriers of a higher-peace conscious nature that honors the health-sustaining energies of the garden-culture food supply, fueled by earth, wind, rain and sun.

Archaeologists have thought for a while that most settled ancient populations survived on a vegetarian diet and now carbon isotope analysis has given experts a better idea than ever before of what the ancient Egyptians ate… The ancient people ate mostly 'C3' plants such as garlic, aubergines, pears, lentils and wheat…*KRIST Text*, p.119

Let raw and living fruits, vegetables, seeds, nuts, herbs and spice be your healing source.

We are talking about the holistic living healing properties of herbs and let us not let forget the magnificent aromatherapy of those plants that we call spice.

CODE GREEN: HIDDEN POWERS OF THE GARDEN TARGETING THE IMMUNE SYSTEM

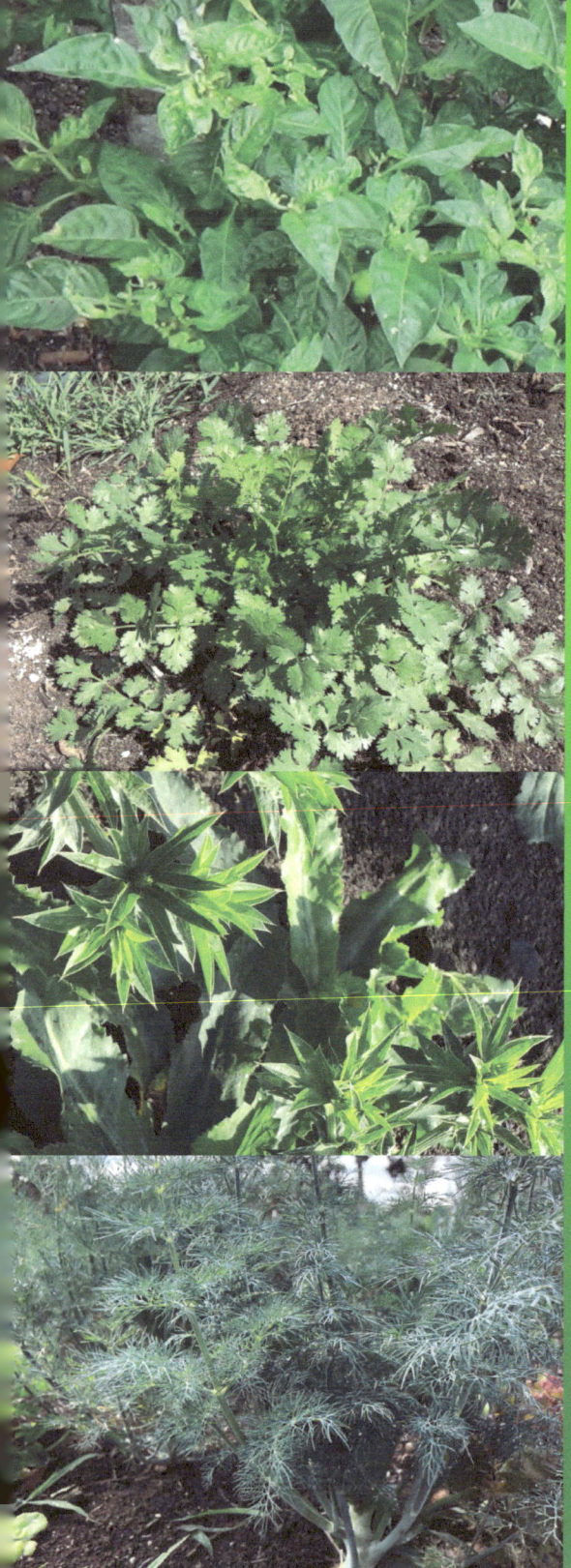

Basil tops the list for foods with Vitamin K, which plays a role in blood clotting and bone strengthening. It contains high beta-carotene, vitamin A, which is essential for vision, healthy mucus membranes and skin. It supports the nervous and immune systems.

Cilantro is a beneficial source of vitamins A, B_6, C, E, K and more. Cilantro is reported as increasing antioxidant levels, aiding in heavy metal detoxification, enhancing the immune defense system and liver function, and having anti-inflammatory properties.

Culantro has been used traditionally to treat a number of ailments. It is high in vitamins A, B and C — all of which are potent antioxidants that help promote vitality and immunity.

Dill contains vitamin A, an essential nutrient important for maintaining vision and supporting a healthy immune defense system. Dill also contains vitamin C which is vital to the immune system and helps with bone formation, wound healing and metabolism.

CHAPTER 8: HERBAL DEFENSE -- CULINARY CONDIMENTS

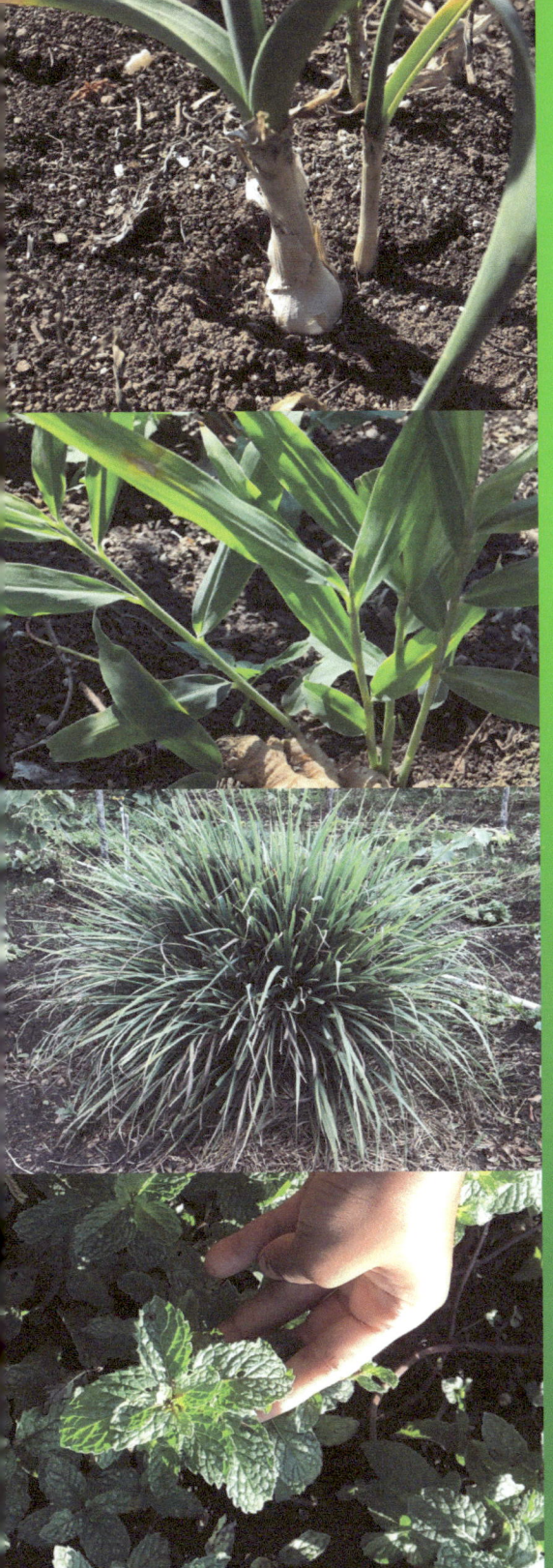

Garlic contains the immune-stimulating compound allicin which promotes the activity of white blood cells to destroy certain viruses. It has noted anti-viral, anti-inflammatory, and anti-fungal benefits. Eat it raw for medicinal effects.

Ginger has long been used to protect and promote a healthy digestive system. Ginger is also effective in reducing fever and easing pain, and it is noted as a powerful anti-bacterial and anti-viral agent.

Lemongrass is recognized as an effective herb that is used to address insomnia, stomach and respiratory disorders, fever and infection. It is noted as having strong anti-bacterial, anti-fungal and antiseptic properties. The antioxidant activity of lemongrass boosts immune system function.

Mint has antioxidants that increase circulation, allowing white blood cells to increase the speed of defending against viruses and bacteria. Menthol from mint has a relaxing effect that can ease stress and allow the immune system to function properly.

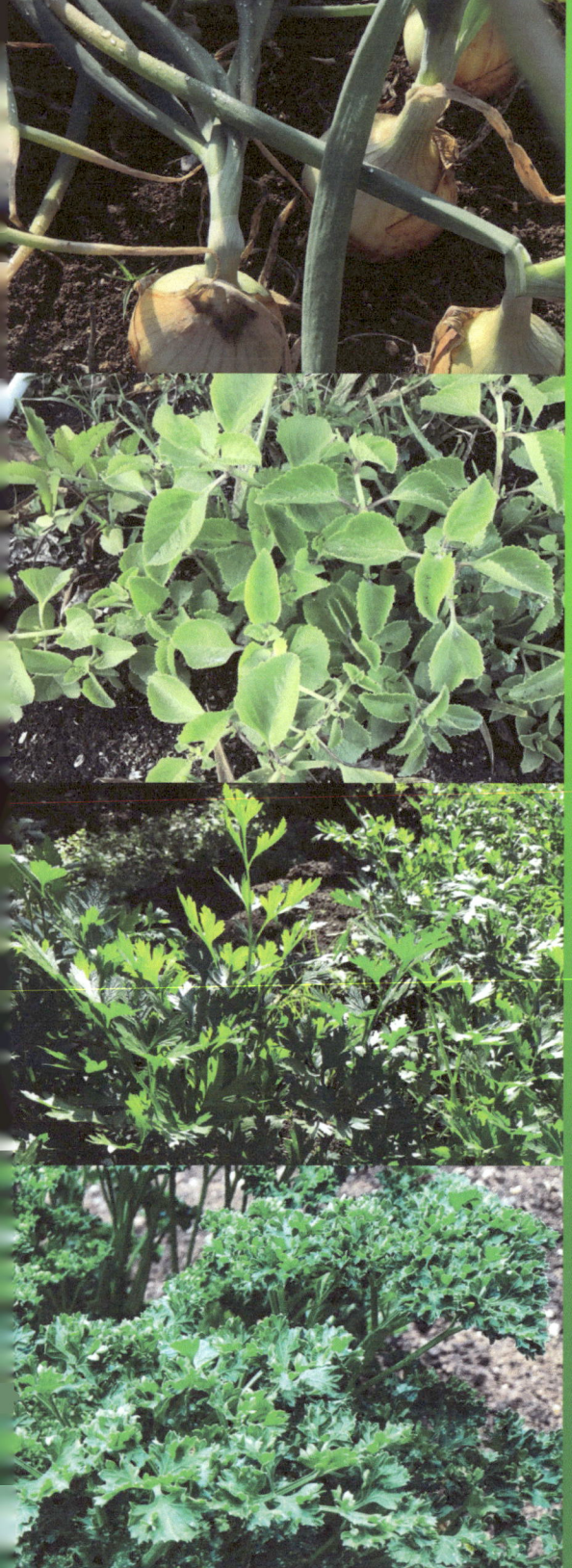

Onion contains quercetin, a nutrient that breaks up mucous strengthening the immune defense system. Onions also contain allicin which is reported to slow down and eliminate a variety of pathogens. Research indicates that consuming raw onion provides immune support within a few hours.

Oregano, bush variety, is used for culinary and medicinal purposes and is reported to be an excellent anti-septic, anti-fungal, anti-bacterial, and anti-spasmodic. It is also said to be a beneficial treatment for chronic coughs, fevers, indigestion and painful swellings.

Parsley, flat and curly leaf, is an excellent source of vitamin C and a good source of vitamin A through its concentration of beta-carotene. Since vitamins A and C are needed for the healthy function of the immune system, parsley can also be helpful for preventing infections.

CHAPTER 8: HERBAL DEFENSE -- CULINARY CONDIMENTS

Peppers, Cayenne family — African Bird pepper, cayenne, habanero, Scotch bonnet, etc.) contain capsicum, a rich source of vitamin C and bioflavinoids that aid your immune system. These help the body produce white blood cells, essential to the lymphatic system to cleanse the cells and tissues of toxins.

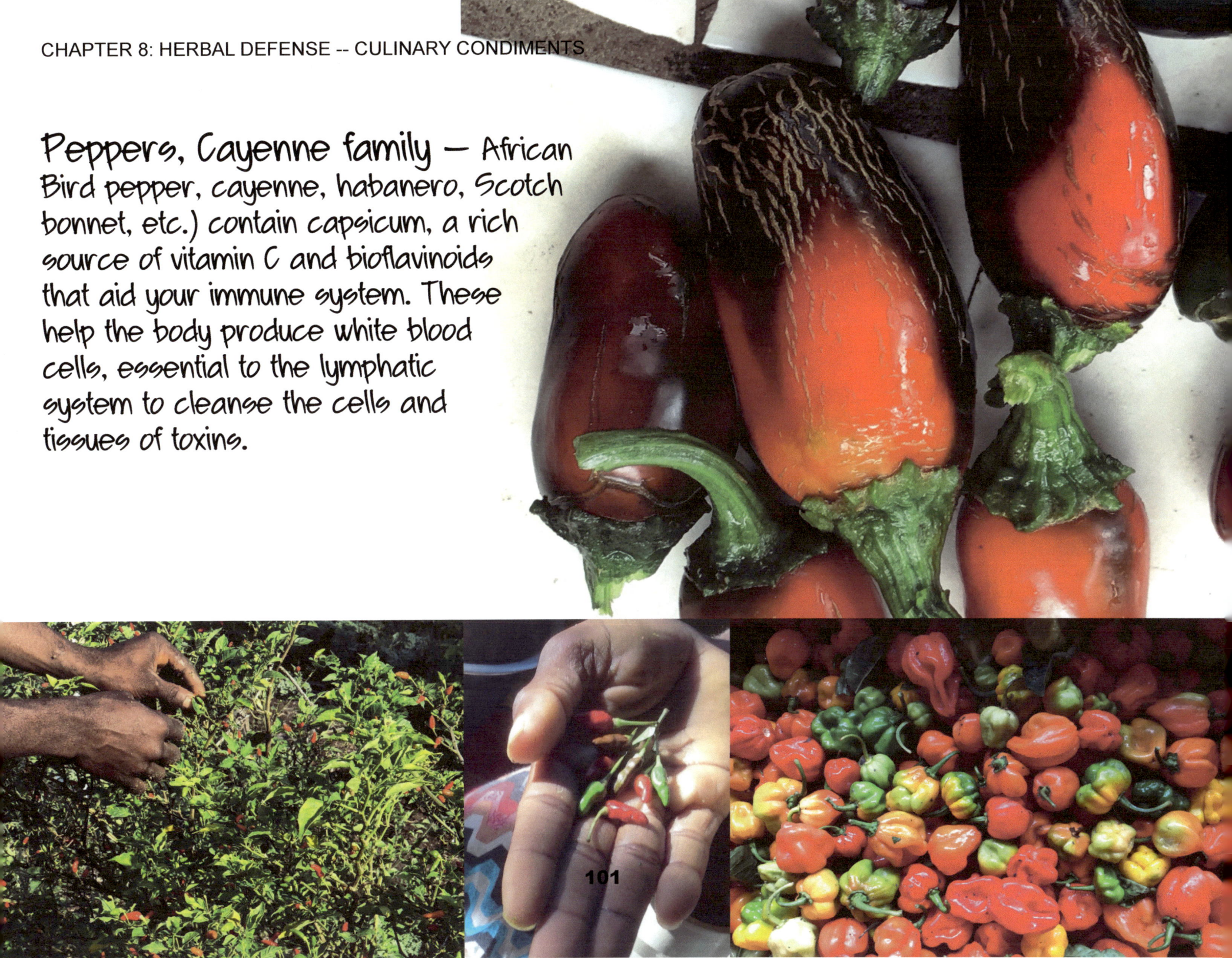

CODE GREEN: HIDDEN POWERS OF THE GARDEN TARGETING THE IMMUNE SYSTEM

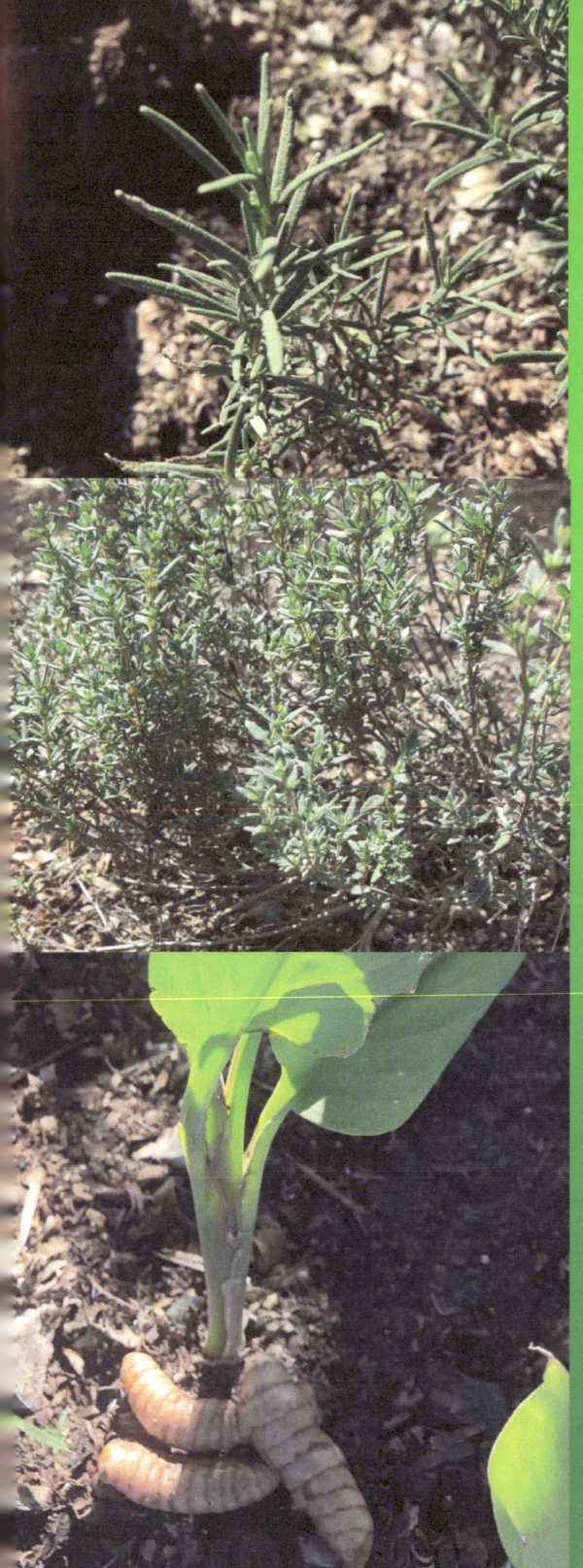

Rosemary is a good source of iron, calcium, and vitamins A, C and B_6. Rosemary has been used for its healing benefits for centuries. Rosemary is rich in antioxidants and anti-inflammatory compounds which are reported to enhance the immune system and improve circulation as it helps detoxify the blood.

Thyme has a long history in being used to support the immune defense system and the mucus membranes. It is known to be an immune system stimulant and a powerful antiseptic against bacteria, viruses, fungi, etc. Thyme helps to fight infection, revitalize, purify the intestines and strengthen immunity.

Turmeric has a bright gold color mainly from circumin, a compound that researchers have identified as having anti-inflammatory, anti-viral, anti-bacterial, and anti-fungal abilities. Studies show that turmeric acts as an antioxidant as well. Circumin has been found to improve antibody response.

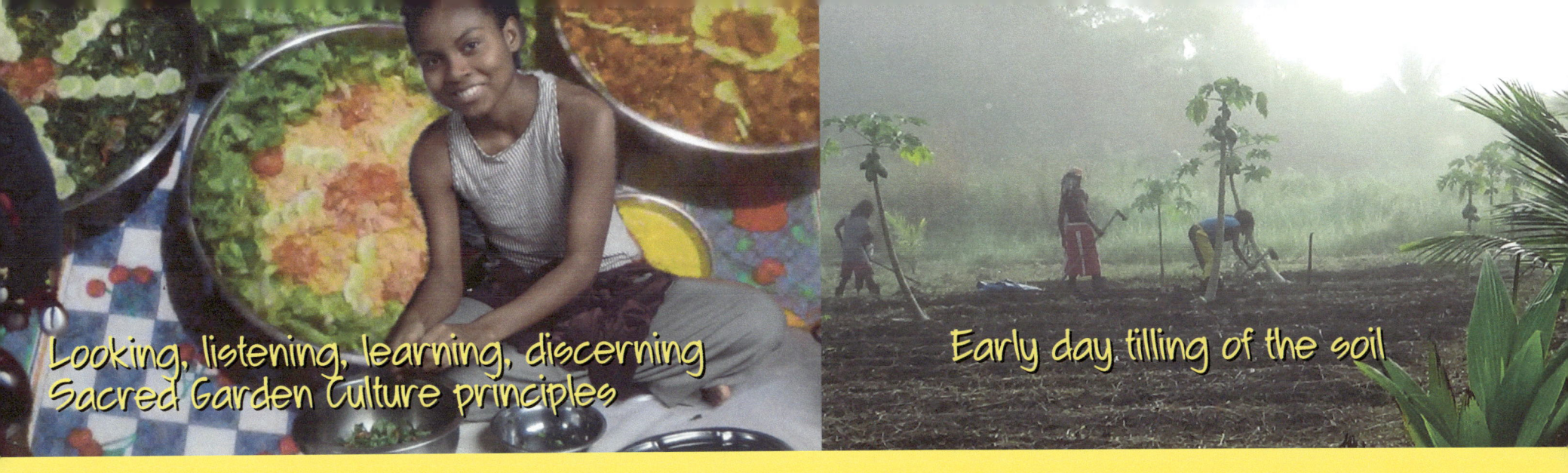

Looking, listening, learning, discerning Sacred Garden Culture principles

Early day tilling of the soil

Reciprocation

A primary law of comprehension within the Kwatamani First Genesis Tribe is the divine law of reciprocation. We say again: what you put in is what will come out and that is what will come back to you again and again. All of the men, women and children within divine social-economic family-community order are aware that food scraps or leftovers, tree clippings, leaves and other natural organic matter are to be gathered and broken down into compost used to fertilize the soil. We have learned that practicing this kind of natural caring and loving soil cultivation forwards a reciprocating relationship with Mother Earth and produces a bountiful, nutrient-rich harvest, infused with natural caring and loving energies.

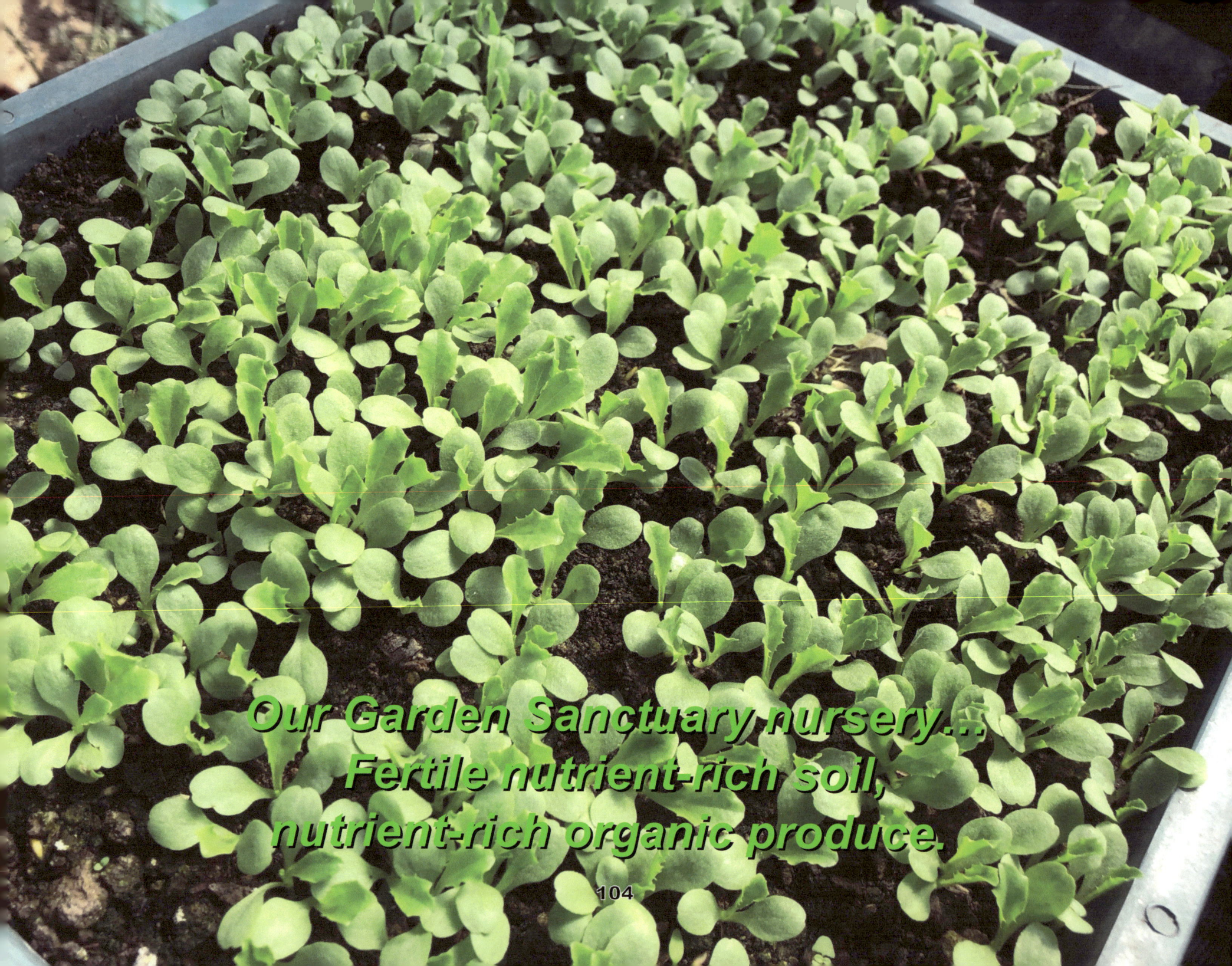

Our Garden Sanctuary nursery... Fertile nutrient-rich soil, nutrient-rich organic produce.

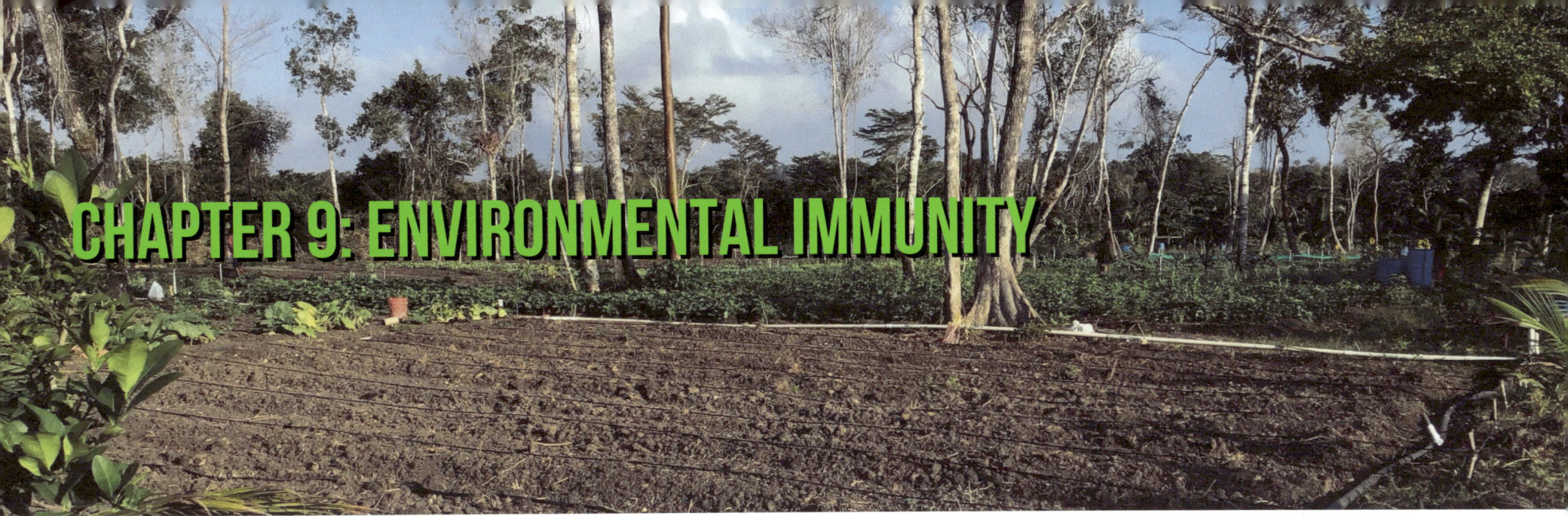

CHAPTER 9: ENVIRONMENTAL IMMUNITY

A quick health check for humanity reveals that mass populations are suffering from a weak and depleted immune defense system. The collective body of Man, He and She, has been invaded by the chronic conditions of sickness and disease, mental disorders and social ills. Conflict, confusion and chaotic destruction…are symptoms and signs of the toxic infection of a debilitating nature of thought, reasoning and action. Indeed, this infection is spreading like a viral plague. And the worse case scenario shows that those who are victims of this plague have been so adversely affected that most will sit and do little or nothing while aiding in their own demise by continuing to indulge in the same toxic attitudes, values, behaviors and beliefs over and over again, hoping and praying for relief.

In our natural state, the immune defense system protects the personal body against the attack and invasion of harmful substances and requires nutritional support to fuel the optimum functioning of that system. In general terms, wholesome health is a natural and innate state of being and must be fueled by a nature of energy that is able to sustain the harmony and balance of all body systems working together in wholeness.

CODE GREEN: HIDDEN POWERS OF THE GARDEN TARGETING THE IMMUNE SYSTEM

Truth or Consequences

In fact, wholeness is defined as "good mental and physical health" and well-being. We refer to the life-sustaining nature of energy that fuels wholeness as whole life energy.

Depleting and Devitalizing

As most people would agree, one can choose to eat food substances that support the health of the body or one can eat food substances for self-satisfaction to indulge in appetites that deplete and destabilize the health of body systems, weakening the immune system and decreasing the body's ability to defend against infections and disease. We refer to depleting and destabilizing food substances as fuel of an opposition energy, because what is consumed actually serves to oppose – that is, to deplete and devitalize – one's natural and innate state of wholesome health and well-being.

Thus, when opposition energy is consumed as dead, devitalized and depleted food substances over a period of time, one will suffer from health problems. For example, over-cooking or any process that alters the natural state of the food, chemical additives, preservatives, MSG, saturated fats, refined sugars, excessive salt, and artificial colors, tastes, and smells do indeed degrade and denature the nutrient quality of the food. As a

CHAPTER 9: ENVIRONMENTAL IMMMUNITY

result, consuming of such degraded and denatured food substances can upset the digestive system, disrupt the nervous system, weaken the immune defense system, and cause serious nutritional deficiencies over time. When this occurs, signs and symptoms begin to show clearly that one is in a state of failing health. By failing health, we are identifying those debilitating physical or mental conditions, such as diabetes, high blood pressure, low blood pressure, heart attacks, cancer, chronic infections, obesity, anxiety, depression, stress and the list goes on and on.

On a larger scale, it is difficult to ignore the signs of failing health that have befallen the collective body of humanity. While there are so many opinions and theories about what is ailing so many people, we state simply that one is a sum total of the nature of energy that one consumes, mentally, physically and spiritually. Regardless of what one claims, the nature of energy that one consumes can only provide fuel to perpetuate that same nature, again and again.

Therefore, unhealthy, degrading and depleted fuel perpetuates cells, organs, tissues, and systems that

stress

DIABETES

ANXIETY

???

heart attack

produce an unhealthy, degraded and depleted state of being. And this unhealthy, degraded and depleted state of being produces an unhealthy, degraded and depleted state of mind. And such an unhealthy state of mind can only produce thoughts, reasoning and actions that will perpetuate unwholesome, unhealthy and depleted attitudes, values, behaviors and beliefs.

If we are clear up to this point, one can see that the nature of fuel one consumes will manifest either a healthy or unhealthy state of being. The signs and symptoms of sickness, disease, infection and disorder signal a warning to return to a natural and innate state of health and well-being, or continue down a road of self-destruction. Self-destruction, that is, the whims and wants of Self stand opposed to the orderly requirements for maintaining a wholesome and healthy state of being, and this opposition accelerates the destructive decline of one's brain, body and spirit. Such is the case with the body of humanity, regardless of race, creed, color, sex or national origin.

While whole life energy fuels a holistic living nature that promotes wholesome health and well-being, the opposition energy fuels an intrusive, invasive warlike nature that promotes death and deadly destruction as the tools of its survival. We have seen the damage caused by the warlike nature, a nature of invasion, conquest and

DEGRADED

unhealthy

UNWHOLESOME

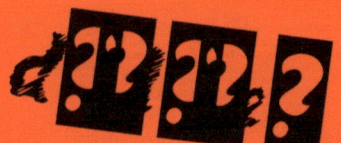

CHAPTER 9: ENVIRONMENTAL IMMMUNITY

Hunting, Herding, War Culture

enslavement that has been waged against the collective body of humanity like a viral plague.

The hunting, herding and war culture survives and capitalizes on blood spill, feasting on the flesh of the prey, and glorifying in the thrill of the kill as victory. Social, economic, political and religious systems fueled by this divisive, opposition nature of energy can only produce a food supply that fuels this same nature of Self as it seeks the ways and means of death and deadly destruction. We must never forget that one is a sum total of the nature of energy that one consumes, mentally, physically and spiritually. Thus, a dead, devitalized and depleted fueling source has no alternative except to perpetuate attitudes, values, behaviors and beliefs that fuel sexual violation, violence, war and crime.

Remember here that invasive pathogens attack and infect the body to target, occupy and destroy healthy cells, and remember the role of the immune defense system is to protect the integrity of a healthy body.

First Genesis

And remember that we are speaking from the holistic living consciousness of the Kwatamani First Genesis Tribe. As such, we are in an on-going, working alignment with the First Genesis of humanity as preserved ages ago in oral traditions of sacred elders within the Kemetic Naga Priesthood. These teachings were later revived and kept alive by a Kemetic priesthood initiate named Moses. The First Genesis has been strategically placed and secured through time by the Most Supreme Unseen Essence of Masculine and Feminine energy:

Genesis 1: 26–30

Then God said, "Let us make mankind in our image, in our likeness…So God created mankind in his own image, in the image of God he created them; male and female he created them. God blessed them and said to them, "Be fruitful and increase in number…Then God said, "I give you every seed-bearing plant on the face of the whole earth and every tree that has fruit with seed in it. They will be yours for food…And to all the beasts of the earth and all the birds in the sky and all the creatures that move along the ground – everything that has the breath of life in it–I give every green plant for food. And it was so."

The principles of the First Genesis are re-encoded in these times through the Most Supreme Unseen Essence of the Kemetic Naga

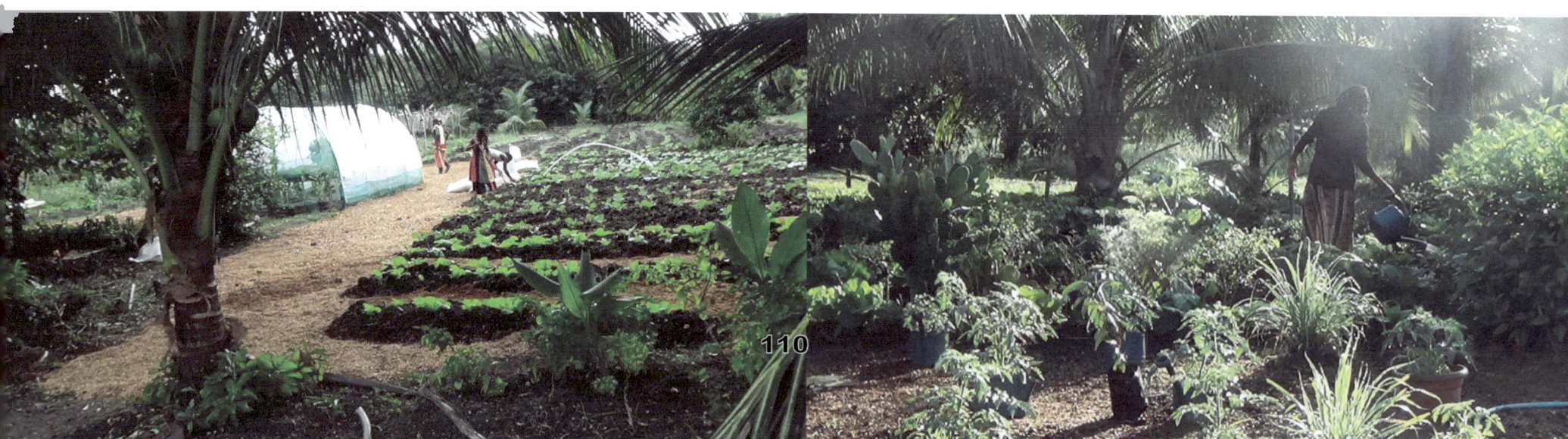

CHAPTER 9: ENVIRONMENTAL IMMMUNITY

Priesthood, transmitted through the Sacred Ancestral Temple of Kwa-Ta-Man-I. "In the beginning, the Most Supreme Unseen said, 'Let us make man in our own image, us not I, our not my, and so it was and so it came to be…divine union, He and She, holistically.'" Thus, the Most Supreme Essence of who we be, He and She, forwards the Sacred Order of the Ankh, the key to holistic living healing.

- Divine Consumption, raw and living fruits, vegetables, seeds, nuts, herbs and spice from the Tree of Life

- Divine Union of masculine and feminine energy, He and She

- Forward Multiplication of Divinity into every offspringing vibration of the Generation Next through divine social economic family community order

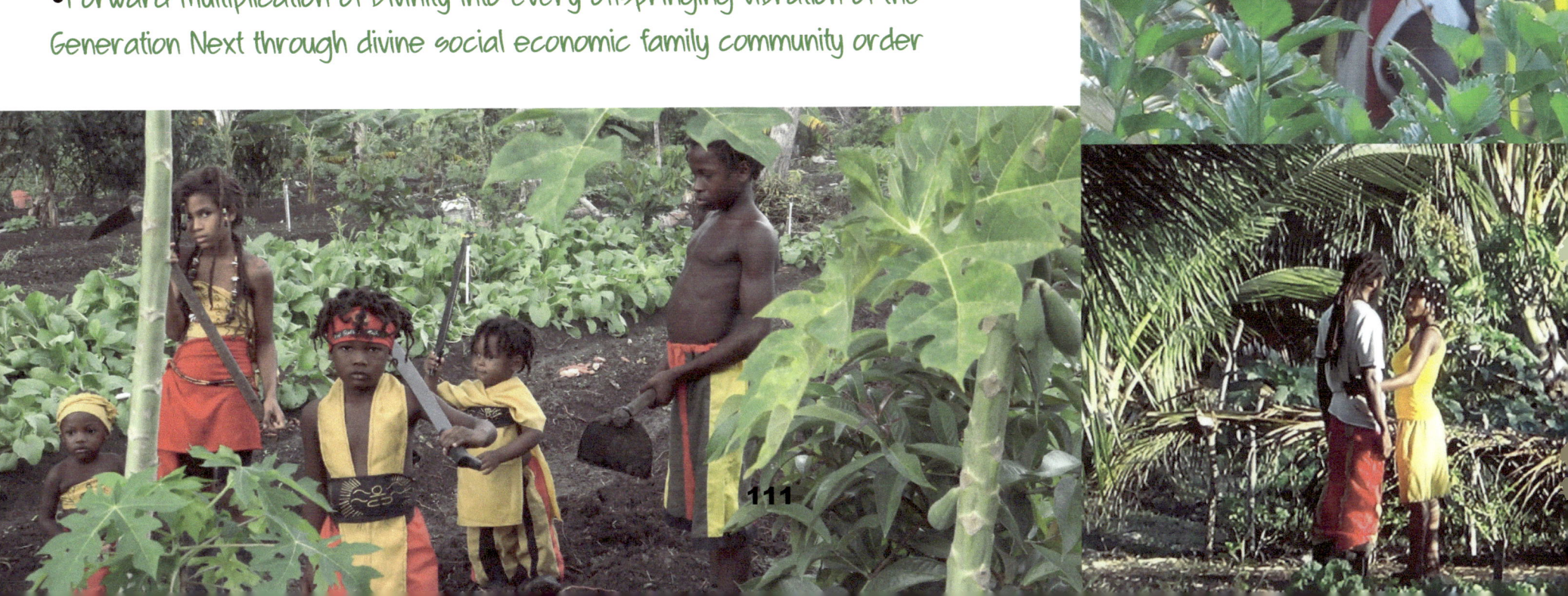

Consider that this Supreme Truth states the universal principles necessary to sustain humanity's existence which are needed now more than ever before. We are talking about the body of Man, He and She, at this time upon Mother Earth. Our collective body as a global family community of humanity who share the same vital resources of earth, wind, rain and sun. Ours is not to horde the natural resources that fuel our existence and supply our basic needs while mass populations starve and suffer and perish in despair. Ours is not to violate and rape Mother Earth, stripping her bare, polluting and defiling her magnificent nurturing bounty. Ours is not to honor a war culture as it feeds upon an opposition energy that glorifies he who has the swiftest ability to kill, maim, conquer and destroy.

Ours is to strengthen our natural and innate immune defense system to eliminate the pathogenic presence of a viral plague that has infected the consciousness of so many. We are talking about a mental plague that perpetuates the viciously divisive profiles of race, sex, and religion to divide, conquer and rule over humanity, Mother Earth and all living things thereof; a plague of self-asserted

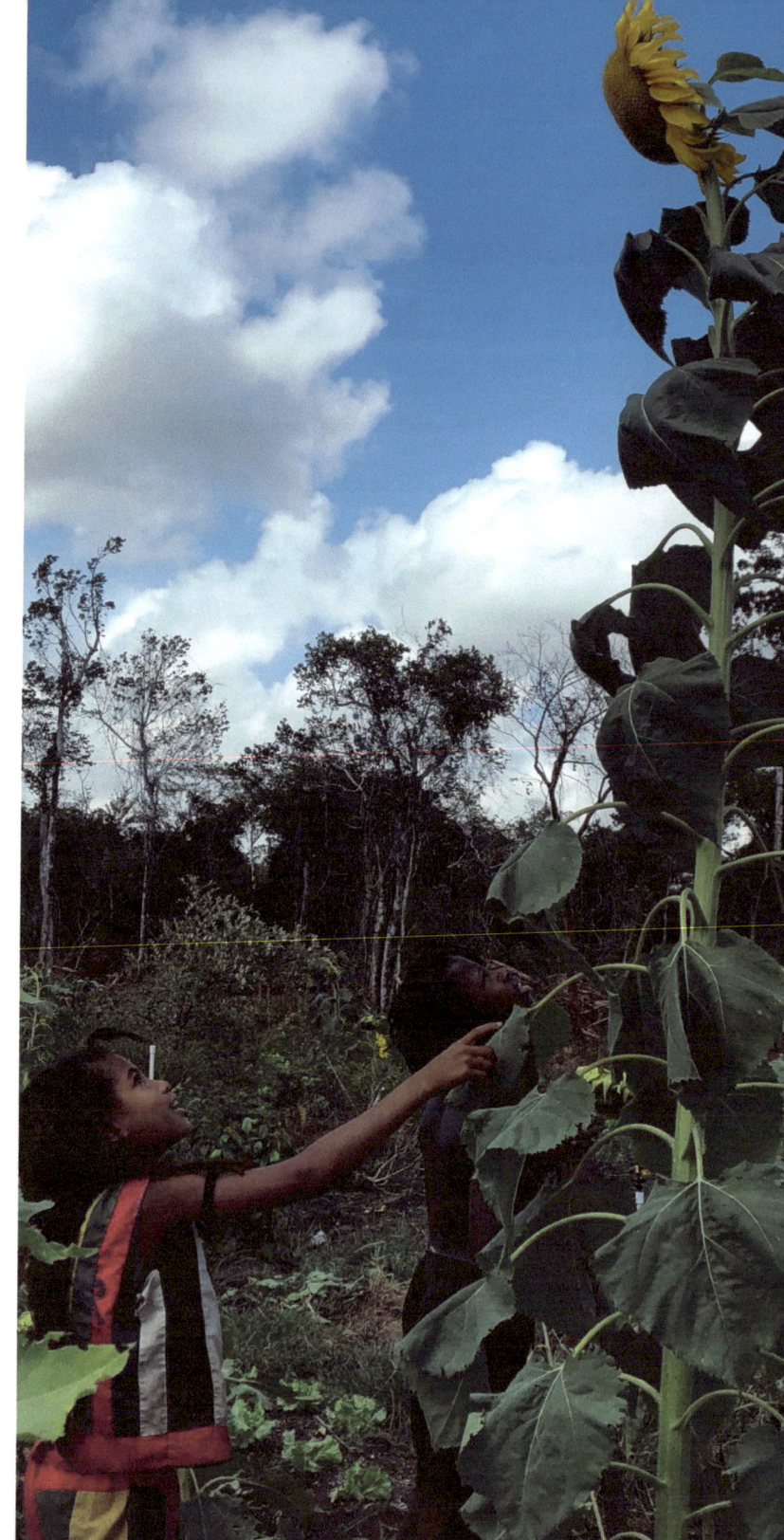

CHAPTER 9: ENVIRONMENTAL IMMMUNITY

individualism, a plague of monotheistic supremacy that opposes the divine union of masculine and feminine energy, and thereby opposes the wholeness of our existence as Man, He and She. Our natural and innate immune defense system functions to de-tox, purge and heal as the pathway to wholeness, that is, the pathway to collective wholesome health and well-being.

De-toxing secures the wholeness and integrity of the body through a systematic process of elimination to neutralize the adverse effects of any harmful invasive presence. This may better explain why we state, "De-tox, purge and heal from the toxic ordeals of the self-asserted, individualistic will".

Alert

Current circumstances facing global populations at this critical time cause the I in I to conclude our text right here. There has been an urgent call for the information presented.

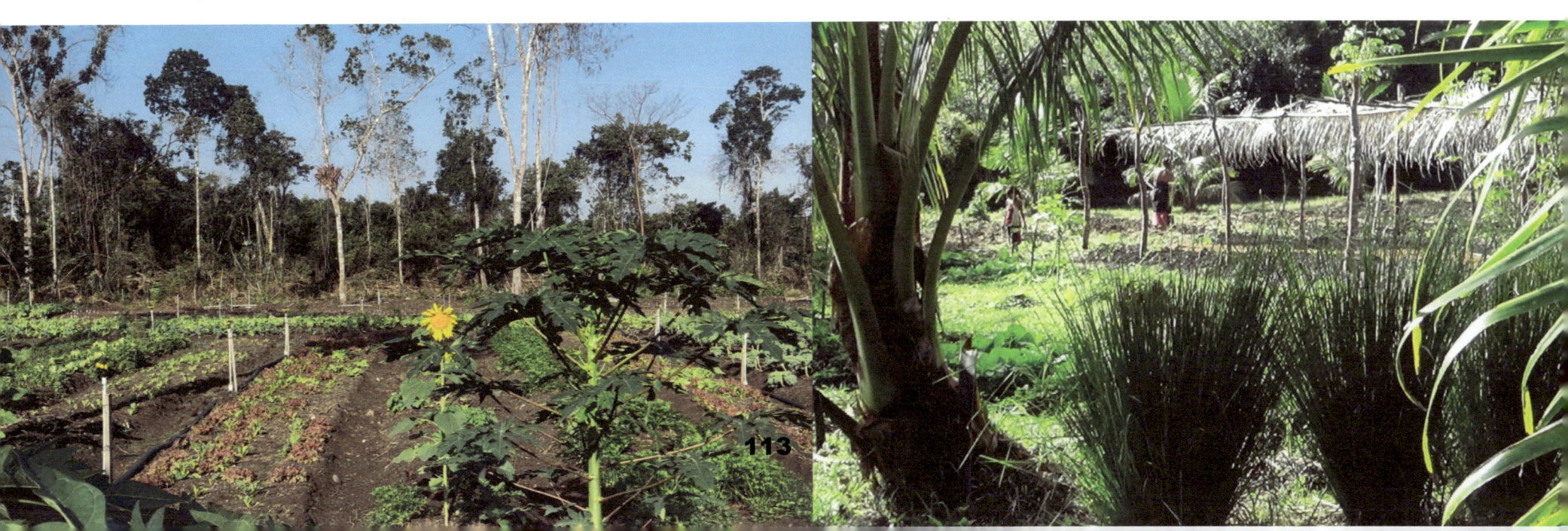

Closing Song: "A New Day Has Begun"

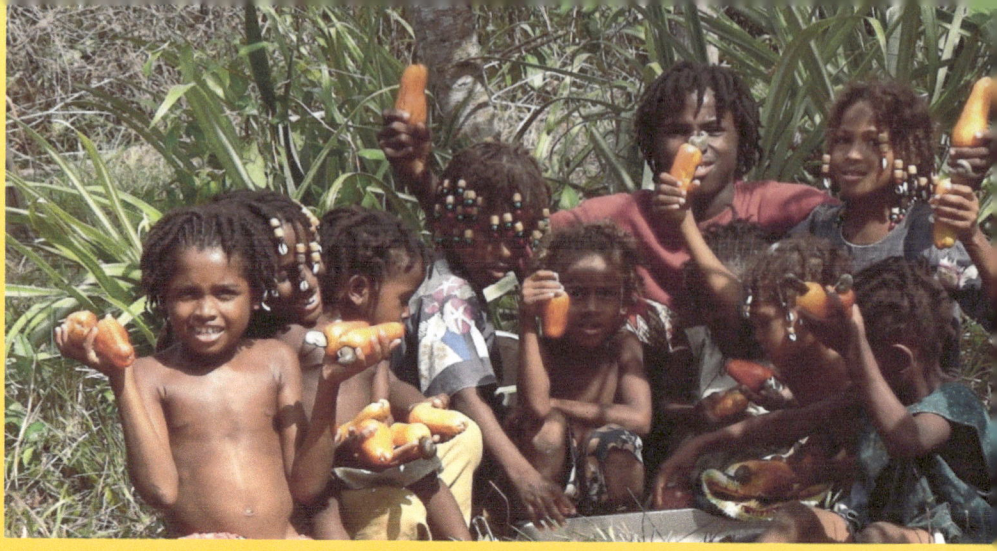

Yeah, it's a new day

Masculine and feminine energy, Most Supreme
nothing less than giving us this opportunity to
resurrect the Sacred Garden Culture of the He
and She of Man, The Most Supreme Master Plan,

Although time would show that most do not
know what this birth meant
Time would show that the I in I was sent, seen and
unseen,
to resurrect ancestral Naga consciousness whole
and clean
Divine spirit consciousness, if you do not know
what I mean
Critical time, much would be revealed
Much did I see, sense, hear, taste and feel

Yet, until the triple-nine gathering time, the inner I
lip was sealed
In the midst of this critical time

The I in I was given instructions to find
A rain forest jungle land divine
Critical time, no time to debate
Critical time no time to hesitate
Critical time for divine social-economic family-
community fate

Critical time to relocate off the grid, natural and
innate
As the weight of self-centered insanity
moving to a more critical state, pale vanity
From a child to grown, the I in I was shown
All that the ancestors had known
About the death culture and how it did begin
And how it was coming to its pathetic end
Danger sign, spirit body and mind on a fatal
decline

Sexual violation, violence war and crime
Guided and protected by the monotheistic mind
In the midst, the I in I was instructed to stand firm
Teaching all that the I in I did learn

True preparation for the New Benu
Providing an exit, a rescue for a Sacred Few
who do seek to find their way through
the rot and the stank and the funk and the smell
Hidden behind the pale veil of the toxic parallel
The I in I would have to go deep within
Far beyond dividing lines of race, class and skin
Far beyond where any Self has ever been
Staying deep in the flow
Guiding divine social-economic family-
community order, watching it grow

Just as the I in I had been shown
All that the ancestors have known

High Priest Kwatamani Truth Lyrics Rap Release Date 2014

As it was in the beginning,
Children of the Sun
A new day has begun...
Ain't nothing like a Naga with an attitude, Hey....

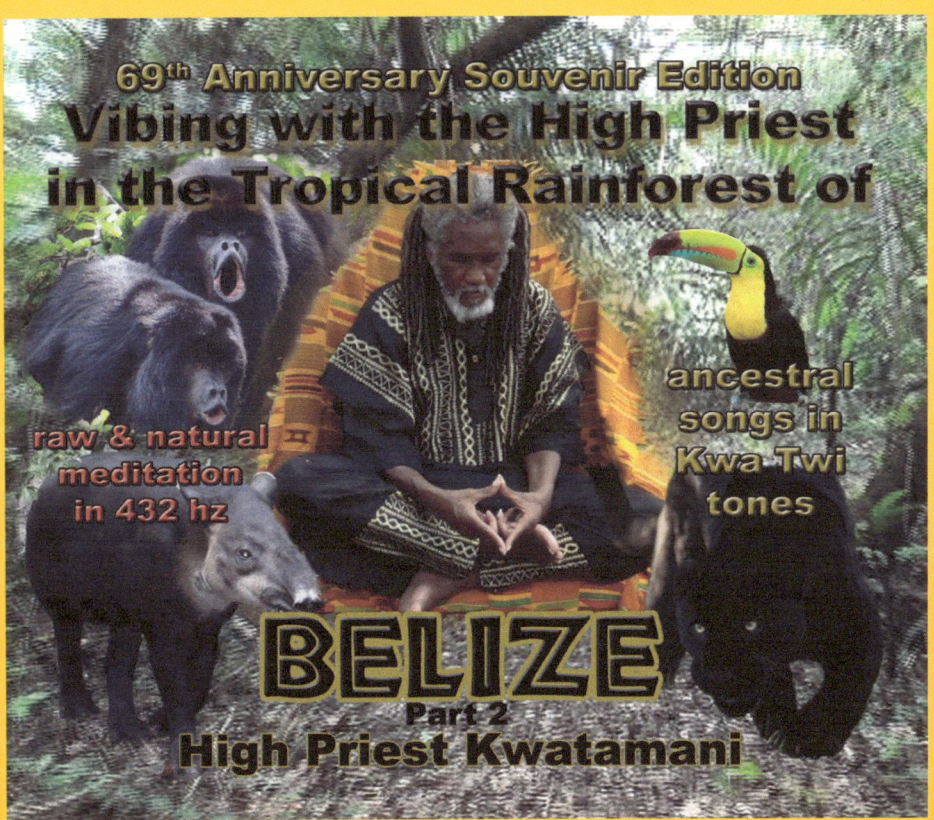

www.ingramcontent.com/pod-product-compliance
Lightning Source LLC
Chambersburg PA
CBHW041327290426

44110CB00005B/159